T0246289

DARE I SAY IT

DARE I SAY IT

EVERYTHING I WISH
I'D KNOWN
ABOUT MENOPAUSE

Naomi Watts

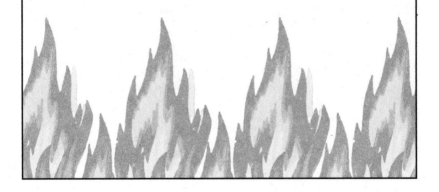

CROWN
NEW YORK

Crown
An imprint of the Crown Publishing Group
A division of Penguin Random House LLC
crownpublishing.com

ISBN 978-0-593-72903-8
Ebook ISBN 978-0-593-72904-5

Library of Congress Cataloging-in-Publication Data
LC record available at https://lccn.loc.gov/2024028912
LC ebook record available at https://lccn.loc.gov/2024028913

Editor: Gillian Blake
Editorial assistant: Amy Li
Production editor: Terry Deal
Jacket designer: Christopher Brand
Text designer: Andrea Lau
Production manager: Heather Williamson
Copy editor: Susan M. S. Brown
Proofreaders: Jill Twist and Carla Benton
Indexer: Elise Hess
Publicist: Tammy Blake
Marketer: Kimberly Lew
Interior art credits: (*megaphone*) © Eleonora Galli/Getty Images; (*flames*) CSA Images/Getty Images

Manufactured in the United States of America

9 8 7 6 5 4 3 2 1

First Edition

For the generations of women who've suffered in silence.

And for the next generations, may they suffer no more.

CONTENTS

CHAPTER FIVE

Will I ever feel like myself again? Should I take
antidepressants? Is it normal to be so anxious? Why do I
want to *throw something*?

CHAPTER SIX

What is hormone therapy, and is taking it a good idea for
me? What do menopause doctors mean when they talk
about "the study"?

CHAPTER SEVEN

What should I know about delivery methods and dosages
and how long to be on hormone therapy?

CHAPTER EIGHT

Is it brain fog or Alzheimer's? How can I improve my memory?

CHAPTER NINE

Why is my skin so dry? Should I get Botox? Do I really need
eighteen serums?

CHAPTER TEN

Why am I waking up all the time? What should I do about
night sweats? Does alcohol really compromise sleep? Will I
ever feel well rested again?

CHAPTER SIXTEEN

What are the biggest health risks at this age? What tests
should I be getting? How should I talk to my doctor about
hormones and everything else?

CHAPTER SEVENTEEN

How can I find meaning and give back? What's the
good news?

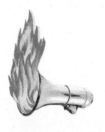

FOREWORD

by Mary Claire Haver, MD

I first met Naomi Watts when I was invited as a medical expert to collaborate on the launch of Stripes Beauty, her company offering products and education to support women during menopause. At the time, I had been exclusively treating menopausal patients out of my own clinic for about eighteen months. I'd become aware that women were increasingly seeking out self-care treatments to address the distinct changes they were noticing in their bodies. I had always admired Naomi's work as an actor, and I was intrigued by her idea to help address the needs of her contemporaries. And now I am honored to introduce you to her marvelous and important book!

In person, I've found her to be wonderfully open to sharing her own story of early menopause and fertility challenges. These experiences fueled her desire to build a community so that other women need not be blindsided by such experiences. She believes, as do I, that we shouldn't be left helpless in dealing with the challenges of the menopausal transition. I've always appreciated the fact that she wasn't interested in selling menopause "cures" (which don't exist), and instead was focused on conveying whatever information she's found useful herself and compassionately supporting other women.

When, in 2022, Naomi began collaborating on menopause symposiums with The Swell, a midlife community designed to help women reimagine how they age, I was thrilled to connect in person with an eager and interested audience of menopausal women. These gatherings also helped me learn a tremendous amount about myself, granted me access to advancements in science and menopause care, and led me to a tribe of like-minded physicians—now known as "the menoposse"—who are revolutionizing how we treat, study, and conceptualize menopause.

The movement to overhaul menopause gained momentum thanks in large part to women like Naomi who were brave enough to stand up and say, "I'm no longer going to be silent about my experience." For her, speaking out as a famous Hollywood actress had the additional risk of being ostracized by the entertainment industry, a space that routinely shelves women who are open about the complexities of aging while female. But it had the additional benefit, for us, of using her glamour to help remove the stigma around menopause, and even making it seem cool.

For many women, the menopausal transition and menopause itself bring about unexpected changes to everything from skin tone and hair quality to sexual health to matters of mood and memory. What the woman in mid- (and mid-ish) life needs when facing these issues is support, which may come in the form of a doctor who finally listens or a friend who's going through the same thing. By being honest about her own and her friends' experiences in dealing with the shock of menopause, Naomi offers validation to other women and makes them feel less alone.

But she goes even further in her effort to help. For *Dare I Say It,* Naomi consulted a number of the top menopause experts in the country. Their clinical perspectives smartly support the lived experiences of women in the menopausal transition and provide practical advice, too.

For years, Naomi has been sharing her story and her knowledge in symposia and among peers. With *Dare I Say It,* her bravery, honesty, and humor will provide much-needed solace and encouragement to an even wider circle. I applaud Naomi dedicating these pages to such a candid telling of her own experience and to sharing so much profound wisdom and useful guidance. This is a great gift to the community of menopause education!

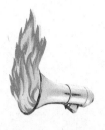

INTRODUCTION

What Is Menopause?

"Looks like you're close to menopause," my doctor told me when I was thirty-six and wondering why I was having so much trouble getting pregnant.

I almost fell off the examination table.

"What do you mean?" I said, gasping for air. "Close to *meno-pause*? That's for grandmothers! I'm not even a mother yet! And, by the way, that's what I'm here for, to become a mother! Take it back!" I was trying to joke, but really I was begging him to make it not be true. I was so scared that this would be the end of my dream to bear children.

As I sat there stunned and full of self-recrimination, I remembered that my mother had once mentioned she'd hit menopause at forty-five—but forty-five still felt very far away from thirty-six. And, frankly, I didn't even really know what menopause meant—except very likely the conclusion of my acting career, which got underway far later than most. When I'd hit my early thirties, people had started telling me that the time would soon come when I wouldn't be able to play a leading lady anymore. Was this the end that had been foretold? I begged the doctor for more information.

He explained that technically menopause is a single day, when you've gone one full year since your last period. This happens on average at the age of fifty-one, and for years leading up to menopause—in the phase now known as "perimenopause"—you can experience a host of symptoms connected with declining estrogen: night sweats, unpredictable periods, mood swings, and weight gain being among the most common. (Shoutout to the relatively recent rise in the use of the term "perimenopause," which according to the OED entered the lexicon in the early 1930s; "menopause" was named way back in 1821 by a French doctor named Charles-Pierre-Louis de Gardanne; it was about time for an expansion of our vocabulary!)

I'd been having night sweats for a while, but no doctors—and I'd seen plenty of doctors, because you have to get a physical exam every time you start a new film—had ever made much of them. You know when you go to a doctor's office and you get the lists with a hundred questions? I ticked "night sweats" every time, for years. Each time they were chalked up to stress, or premenstrual syndrome, or an allergic reaction to something I ate or drank—maybe sulfites in wine? And I accepted those explanations. I was often tired or stressed out from demanding shooting schedules or international travel for press junkets.

In my midthirties, my periods started coming close together, sometimes every fifteen to eighteen days. I thought that seemed weird. Still, it never occurred to me that it had anything to do with menopause. But now, sitting there in the doctor's office, I was learning that my irregular periods and night sweats had actually been perimenopausal symptoms, and their cause was not the stress of my overnight shooting schedule or an extra glass of wine with dinner.

The news sank in as I walked out: my periods would be stopping soon, and with them would go any hope of pregnancy. I imagined calling my mother. I'd begin the conversation in a sensitive, loving way, full of warmth and compassion for what she'd endured as a woman of her generation: "What the *hell*, Mum?" Why hadn't she told me more about this inevitable transition?

Eventually, I did get the chance to ask her about how it had been for her.

"My periods fizzled out," she said. "I was emotionally up and down for a long time, had a few years of symptoms, but after forty-five, the periods were all gone, and that was that!"

I expressed shock that I'd gotten so far in life without knowing about any of that.

"I guess these were the conversations I didn't have with you because my mother never had them with me," she said.

How absurd that something so common should be so taboo. And why had I, a relatively worldly person who'd been going to my annual exams and hanging out with the most wonderfully open and fiercely intelligent women my whole life, never once heard "Heads up, here are the details about this thing that's going to happen to you at some point in the coming years and what it might be like"?

Could it be that one reason for the silence around menopause is that women feel like things are just supposed to *hurt*?

Dr. Sharon Malone, a D.C.-based ob-gyn, chief medical officer at Alloy Women's Health and one of the leading menopause practitioners in the country, told me, "I think one of the things that we have got to understand, and study after study has substantiated this, is that we have really normalized suffering as part of womanhood. We suffer from cramps, we suffer in childbirth, we suffer from premenstrual syndrome. These things that exclusively affect women have been understudied across the board. Because the expectation is that women suffer, it is not deemed worthy of redress. Women exaggerate. We're hysterical. *It's all in your head.* This unfortunate perception is still all too common in medicine today. Women still feel they're not heard, they're not seen, and they're not believed. And that's the problem."

The new menopause awareness is helping women get better treatment, but there's still a lot of misinformation out there, and it can be staggering. A few years ago, my children heard me talking about how I was in menopause. I was curious to hear what they'd absorbed about this life stage, so I asked them what they knew. Would they have something to say about making the transition into a powerful new phase of life, about the wise, grounded elders of ancient villages, about how Helen Mirren didn't get famous until she was well into middle age?

"Isn't it when you wet the bed?" said one child.

"It's when old ladies die?" guessed the other child. "Are you dying?"

"No!" I said. Then I thought, *I guess we're all dying, aren't we?* And I started digging myself a hole: "Well, yes, but no, but . . ."

If the story of our fertile lives is an adventure that starts in puberty and ends in menopause, why do so few people talk about the ending to that odyssey and what comes next? Why isn't menopause part of sex education or premarital counseling or any of the conversations preparing us for the coming challenges in life? Even just a quick FYI when you get your first period: "Congratulations! You're starting a journey of fertility during which you may or may not conceive children. Fertility peaks in your twenties and then starts to decline, more rapidly after the age of thirty-five. Your cycle ends on average at fifty-one, maybe much earlier. Be prepared."

So many doctors have since told me that there's an epidemic of misdiagnosing women with everything from fibromyalgia to chronic fatigue to irritable bowel syndrome to clinical depression when, in fact, they were just perimenopausal.

Years ago, I found myself trying to explain all this to a younger friend. With the passion of Cassandra, I warned her not to ignore symptoms or minimize issues with her health, and to rule out menopause before pursuing more obscure tests.

"It's crazy that there's so little information out there!" I ranted to her. "Why do we have to feel like it has to be a secret? Why don't we share everything we've figured out ourselves and find out what worked for other people? Why isn't there some kind of manual?"

"I'd read a book on that," she said. "You should write it."

I resisted her advice for a long time. My fear was too great. Besides, I still knew nothing—just that it was fast approaching, and I was shit scared. I'd been warned ever since I started acting that calling attention to your age—when that age was not twenty-three or younger—would be career suicide. I was told I would never work again if I admitted to being menopausal, or even perimenopausal. Hollywood's lovely term for such women was "unfuckable."

Each year, two million American women enter menopause. That's almost six thousand women a day. We're talking a *billion* menopausal women worldwide. And yet, I felt completely alone. Ignorance of this transition led to shame and fear, and it almost cost me my chance to become a mother. The fact was I'd been showing perimenopause symptoms for some time but had never been told that's what they could be. When a woman comes in complaining of symptoms like night sweats, anxiety, and insomnia, that should be a doctor's cue to make sure she knows the facts about perimenopause and menopause.

I mean, I partly get the doctors' reluctance to open that conversation. After a few years of being in this space and speaking to them one-on-one, I've come to understand how little time they have to strike up a hard conversation. If they have only fifteen minutes with a patient, why would they want to drop a bomb? Surely the messenger would be killed. I would have slapped my own doctor if he hadn't been so bloody handsome! Why not just do the Pap smear or blood test, and if the woman's distraught, hand her a script for an antidepressant or sleeping pill? Punt the menopause conversation to another day and, with any luck, to another doctor!

There's no question that women in their forties and fifties have been gaslit by the medical system, with real consequences to their well-being, even if there's now a welcome pendulum swing toward more attention to menopause and to various forms of symptom relief. And relief is possible! I'll talk about how hormone replacement therapy (also known as HRT, or menopause hormone therapy [MHT], or just hormone therapy [HT]) has helped me, and what questions to ask if you're considering it. I'll use HRT here because that's how it was introduced to me, and I've stuck with it.

I think it's worth considering where the long silence came from.

Might it not have something to do with misogyny, the patriarchy, and ageism? And with our desire not to inconvenience anybody? But why did we women think that should be the goal—to never need any help?

How radical it has been to realize the ways in which I'd silenced myself because of sexism. I've realized that we don't need to people-please. We don't have to make things easy for everyone else at every turn. We can take up space. We can say what we need. We can assert ourselves!

I've also come to believe that there is nothing sexier than a woman who knows what she wants. All good relationships at work and at home—and at the doctor's office—require communication. We can discuss without shame the details of menopause—how to navigate it, what the symptoms could be, and not just "Oh, you might feel warm at some point." But all the *gory details*. I didn't know my skin would get so dry, or that urinary tract infections and GI issues would become commonplace, or that there was such a long list of other issues connected to the menopausal transition. I was craving information on menopause, and certainly no one in Hollywood was breathing a word about it. We were all behaving as if between the seductress years and the grandmother roles, women just . . . I don't know, vanished?

Well, I got madder and madder until I no longer cared about the potential cost to my career. Hell, if I needed information, others probably did, too. And by that point I'd been dealing with menopause for a decade, so I thought that maybe—just maybe—I could offer something to those coming to it fresh.

In October 2022, I founded a company called Stripes Beauty to address various practical needs of women my age (for example, by offering a lubricant "play oil" and an intensive skin moisturizer to help with the massive hydration loss that comes with middle age). Stripes Beauty's three pillars are menopause education, community, and solutions from scalp to vag. In the same spirit, I started working on this book, which will attempt to cover every aspect of menopause I've encountered. It's intended to be the sort of resource I wish I'd had when I walked out of that doctor's office in pieces and truly terrified.

I've written this book for anyone who's going through menopause and trying to figure out what the hell is happening and for everyone who will go through it and wants to be well prepared so that they're not blindsided like I was. I've always shied away from jumping on the soapbox. But the menopause conversation requires us to get honest, loud, and, dare I say it, even a little *unladylike. Faaaaark!*

One of the funniest things that's happened as a result: random celebrities now text me regularly to tell me they're in menopause. It's like I'm behind the confessional window, or I'm Hollywood's agony aunt. But I enjoy it! I welcome them to the club and offer them doctor suggestions or whatever they're looking for, which is often just someone to listen to them without judgment. In this book I'll tell you everything I tell them and in what I hope is enough detail to spare you all the searching I had to do as I was flailing my way through this transition.

Caveat: I'm not a doctor (I've never even really played one in movies, though I played a midwife once), but I've come to know plenty of them since I started banging on about menopause. I've always considered myself someone who's good at putting people together, whether that's throwing a dinner party, producing a film, or organizing a pickleball tournament (yes, I've done that). I trust my instincts when it comes to identifying talented people.

And so that is what I have done here. To offer the most up-to-date information and the most inspiring stories, I've assembled brilliant experts—gynecologists, psychologists, dermatologists—and a diverse group of fascinating women with stories to tell about menopause, from a friend of mine in her seventies having the best sex of her life to a woman in her late forties who had a panic attack live on television.

How do we make this the most empowering, exciting time of

our lives as women? This is when we have the experience in our work, in our relationships, and in our bodies to know what we have to offer the world. We don't need anyone else's permission. All we need are the tools and the information to unapologetically stride into the powerful, joyful age ahead of us.

CHAPTER ONE

DISCOMFORT ZONE

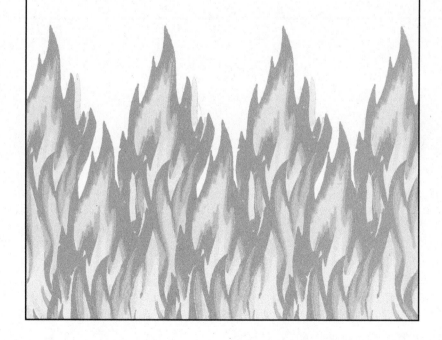

When I was forty-two, not long after my second baby was born, I started having strong, consistent menopause symptoms. My most significant symptom was night sweats. But I had the occasional hot flash during the day, too. I remember two of them distinctly.

One time I was on a plane when a hot flash came on. In that moment, I felt like I was being suffocated. The heat was overwhelming, but the feeling was less like being in a warm climate than like being flooded with shame. I was overcome with the feeling of *Oh my God, I have to get out of here right now!* But I was in a middle seat, and I'd already gotten up for the bathroom a couple of times—much to the chagrin of my seatmate, who'd given me plenty of side-eye looks—so I stayed hunkered down, wishing I could be anywhere else. If there had been an eject button, I would have hit it, right after flipping the bird to the dude in the aisle seat.

Another time, I was taking a fun trip with friends, and we were on a big boat in the Pacific Ocean. It was one of the first times I'd tried to take a glamorous vacation with my toddlers, and I was thrilled to be out on the water in a cute summer outfit. I was suddenly drenched. I barely had any clothes on, but I felt I had to remove even the stringy bits of fabric and dive into the ocean! Even if the boat was moving in shark-infested waters, I thought, *I have to get in the cool water immediately.*

"This was the year the wheels came off," one woman told me about her own experience of realizing that she was entering a new phase of life. While she was having the classic symptoms related to blood vessel dilation and constriction (hot flashes, night sweats, heart palpitations), she started having symptoms in just about every area of her body: mood changes including depression, anxiety, irritability, and rage; skin changes, including somehow both dryness and oiliness; sleep trouble; hair loss on her head coupled rather cruelly with its growth on her face; vaginal dryness and associated sexual problems; loss of libido; migraines; brain fog; UTIs; GI issues; incontinence; and even ringing in the ears. It took her and her doctors a while to realize that they were *all* connected to menopause.

The symptom most strongly associated with menopause is the phenomenon known as "hot flashes," or "hot flushes" in the United Kingdom. (Some doctors in the United States also prefer the term "flush," because the sensation comes on more like an all-over drench than like a lightning strike, but I'm going to stick with "flash" in this book because I've spent the past thirty years in America, so it's what I'm used to.) They can be among the more aggravating issues to deal with at this age, especially because they seem to come on at the least convenient times, since they can be triggered by stress.

My friend Sarah described her hot flashes to me this way: "One weird obsession became shifting my body to one side or another at night and touching the sheet, marveling at how it was as if someone had just removed an electric blanket set to level ten—so incredibly hot to the touch! The biggest surprise for me about hot flashes is how different they feel than just being superhot on a summer day. They are so intense and immediate. I'm feeling fine . . . feeling fine . . . *Oh my God, someone get my fan! Throw ice on me! I don't care if I'm fully nude in public!*" She said this phase of life could be summed up as "ripping one's clothes off while on college tours."

I can't tell you the number of women I've talked to who were in an important meeting at work or having a difficult conversation with a partner and suddenly they found themselves sweating profusely, feeling as though they were in a hot yoga class while everyone else was comfortable as could be. The first time I had a hot flash I thought, *Who turned up the heat? Who is to blame for this?* Like when your pants won't button and you're sure that the machine has shrunk them in the wash.

For me, night sweats were common even though I nearly have to kill myself in an exercise routine before I can work up a sweat. Even now, in spite of hormone therapy, I'll wake with an occasional chest sweat, smelling like I've been flipping burgers in a fast-food joint all night. (Dermatologists have told me that middle-aged women increasingly are showing up in their offices for underarm Botox, which turns off the excessive sweating!)

One of my makeup artists says the first time she ever witnessed a hot flash was at work: "An actress was sitting in my makeup chair and said, 'Oh my gosh, it's coming. It's coming!' I said, 'What are you talking about? What's coming?' And she said, 'Look at my face.' All of a sudden, her skin got really red, and beads of sweat started forming on her upper lip. This was a woman playing a leading lady and wearing sexy clothes. We got her some ice water, and we put cold compresses on her face until she cooled off."

Hot flashes are caused by hormone fluctuation. The body's thermostat gets thrown out of whack by not having the usual amount of estrogen, and so it sends signals saying it's too hot. The body responds by opening up blood vessels, causing sweating and flushing, usually for a few intense minutes.

There are plenty of reasonable things to do to combat hot flashes. Some simple, obvious tips: wear layers so you can strip down quickly when a hot flash starts and use breathable cotton fabrics. Make sure you get sleep and drink water. Monitor your triggers and try not to eat or drink things that bring hot flashes on, like spicy food or alcohol or caffeine (basically everything fun). Chug ice water or put an ice pack on the back of your neck if you feel a hot flash coming. A friend of mine swears by her portable neck fan, which looks like headphones. I know what you're thinking: no ice pack or cute fan is going to save me when I have a hot flash.

"Hot flashes are really just the tip of the iceberg," Dr. Sharon Malone told me. (This is an ironic metaphor; there is nothing cool about them!) "We treat them because we have found that severe and frequent hot flashes are harbingers of an increased risk for cardiovascular disease and can be a risk factor for Alzheimer's disease as well.

"Women with hot flashes have disrupted sleep. Disrupted sleep can lead to more cardiovascular disease, more depression, more irritability, and even weight gain. So while we make jokes about hot flashes and people make light of them, hot flashes are the canaries in the coal mine for other long-term health issues that surface after menopause. And women need to understand that hot flashes are not benign, and they're not funny."

Before I entered menopause myself, I hadn't known that there were any symptoms beyond hot flashes, night sweats, and mood swings. I'd had terrible migraines for years. They would last for three days, right in the same point behind my left eye. Sometimes it would be just a dull ache, but other times it was completely debilitating, and anything could set off a migraine. It didn't always come from an extra glass of wine or too much sugar, though those were reliable triggers. Poor hydration was often the cause, or too little sleep. I was never able to take three days off work and childcare to recover, but if I didn't catch an oncoming migraine with the right meds right away, that's how long it would last. So I would suffer through it. I found these migraines very depressing. And not once in all those years did anyone mention they might be a menopause-related symptom.

Just when I felt like I was getting a handle on migraines, I started getting urinary tract infections, incessantly. The UTIs were causing me to go on antibiotics, which were then causing GI issues—blockages and bloating. I went to the doctor, who said to start using Metamucil and drink lots of water. And that was all the help I was given.

My GP never said, "Well, this is probably related to menopause, and here's what you should do."

So I threw random short-term solutions at the problem. I remembered in my twenties using Ural "urinary alkalinizer" powders from Australia, which make urine less acidic and eliminate some of the burning feeling of UTIs. Now, many years later, I've learned that the powders are available online, even from Amazon, in cranberry or lemon flavors, and so from time to time I order them. But no matter how many products you throw at UTIs, they're still annoying and incredibly painful.

One day during the pandemic, I was in extreme pain from a UTI, and none of the usual drugstore remedies—including cranberry juice, Azo, and Advil—were working. I got in touch with my doctor, who was at a baseball game. (No matter how many telehealth visits I'd had, I couldn't figure out what was going on. I felt like I was being run around in circles, and the doctor was also incredibly hard to reach.) I could barely hear him over the roar of the crowd. He said, "No, it's fine. Just go on this antibiotic, pick it up from the pharmacy and dah, dah, dah."

I put the phone down. It was the fourth course of antibiotics I'd been prescribed in a short period of time. I felt like he was brushing me off, as though I was complaining too much or being a hypochondriac. I thought, *I need help. Isn't it your job to provide it?*

Later, after I gave up on that doctor, I exchanged texts with a new doctor when my face blew up from an allergic reaction to a certain antibiotic. I wasn't sure why it happened, but I suspected either the medication he'd put me on or an environmental factor. My bloodwork showed E. coli, so I sent the doctor a link to an article about a certain kind of dog food that was being linked to that bacteria. (How many of us have turned up the most random articles in our online deep dives?) He wrote back, "Thank you for this interesting article. You might want to get your dog cultured."

With every new round of antibiotics—and my doctor told me they had to keep switching kinds because I'd build up resistance to each one in turn—my stomach would get super bloated. I was in so much pain that finally one doctor sent me for a CT scan. The radiologist told me that my gut was like a filled-up bucket that was about to overflow, and that this state could be extremely dangerous. Essentially, I was about to explode because I was so backed up. *Didn't Elvis die from an exploding stomach?* I thought.

I shake my head as I look back on all those texts with the doctor—"Just stay well hydrated," he said at one point.

In the end, getting help for my chronic UTIs required three doctors, six rounds of antibiotics, one CT scan, multiple enemas, daily Metamucil, a slew of yeast infections from the antibiotics, a bunch of opportunities for intimacy avoided out of fear of discomfort, and a truckload of shame—when all it should have taken was one menopause-savvy doctor and a single tube of estrogen cream!

In those months I was so embarrassed and frustrated. It turned out that GI problems were yet another effect of menopause, which makes a lot of sense given that hormones affect just about everything in your body, including gut bacteria and digestion. Again, there is such poor medical training on menopause. I've heard that, at best, *sometimes* doctors receive four hours of instruction on the subject in their entire residency, perhaps only a single lecture in medical school. No wonder all of us (many doctors included) are at sea.

More menopause-savvy doctors have since said to me that you can take a short-term dose of antibiotics to prevent UTIs, but there are other things that help, too, like peeing before and after sex, and applying estrogen cream a few times a week, plus some extra cream if there may be a roll in the hay ahead. Dryness can be a factor in UTIs and other problems as well.

Dr. Kelly Casperson, a board-certified urologist in the State of Washington, sees patients for what we now call "genitourinary syndrome of menopause," or GSM, formerly called "vulvovaginal symptoms of menopause," or VSM. "But my patients don't know that's what it's called," she said. "What they're coming to me for is 'It's burning when I pee.' 'I'm leaking more.' 'I'm going to the bathroom at work all the time.' Or they complain of recurrent urinary tract infections, or pain with sex, dry vulva, dry vagina.

"And all of those are GSM. With low estrogen, you lose elasticity, and you lose your natural moisture, which is protective to the tissues. We can see these symptoms in perimenopause as well as in older women. And people aren't making the connection. I'll tell a seventy-year-old that her urinary issues are connected to menopause, and she'll say, 'That was fifteen years ago, and I never had hot flashes!' People don't make the connection that the body has certain reactions to low estrogen."

What I've begun to realize, too, is that these symptoms, which seem strictly physical, can reverberate throughout your life. For example, you could suffer the breakdown of a relationship when you're both too scared to have sex because of pain and too embarrassed to speak about it with your partner.

When I described my frequent UTIs, Dr. Casperson said they were common for women my age: "UTIs occur more frequently in midlife as our estrogen levels decline, causing the pH of our vagina to rise. Then our microbiome changes. It's the acidic pH and healthy microbiome of our vagina that helps protect our bladder from the pathogens (or bugs) of our GI tract, which are normal in the GI tract but cause infection when they cross up into the bladder. Think of a healthy vagina like a bouncer at a bar. It works by keeping some things out of the area (GI bugs). With intimacy, fluids get mixed around and that is why bladder infections are more common. So if you want a good party, have a healthy bouncer!"

If you're getting UTIs often, as I was, there are steps you can take. "I tell my patients when I see them for recurrent UTIs—meaning two UTIs within six months or three within a year—that the first thing we have to do is get them out of the cycle of UTIs and antibiotics," says Dr. Casperson. "They get in this cycle of despair because just taking an antibiotic disrupts your microbiome, which makes you more susceptible to getting another UTI. Vaginal estrogen is the answer to break that cycle, and people don't know that." Certainly this could have saved me so much misery!

"People stop having sex because they worry about triggering another UTI. And they get obsessively clean and start using all these products which cause more irritation! We have multiple studies on the role of vaginal estrogen decreasing the recurrence of UTIs—it decreases your risk of UTIs by 50 to 60 percent, which is pretty miraculous." If I'd only known!

The GI stuff has also been such a huge issue for me, and I've only now begun to get it under control. By listening to my body and what works for it, I now recognize when it will help to reduce my intake of things like wheat, caffeine, alcohol, and sugar. Some women have good luck getting their systems in order with high-fiber diets or by taking a probiotic once a day.

Personally, I'm a big believer in moderation. I find sticking to diets exhausting, and the temptation to cheat always gets the better of me. In the past, overusage of supplements has caused me GI issues, so I tend to take them now mainly as correctives when things are feeling out of balance. And I do my best to eat fermented foods like sauerkraut, probiotic yogurt, kombucha, miso, kimchi, and a daily spoonful of apple cider vinegar.

But I've found that hormones have helped me with many of my issues in ways that diet alone didn't. (More on hormone therapy in Chapters 6 and 7.) Dr. Casperson explained: "If you never pee and you're dehydrated and you have a very inflammatory diet, estrogen won't cure everything. Hormone therapy is just part of taking care of yourself. Midlife is really the time to take stock: Are you exercising? Are you trying to have a good diet? Are you managing your stress?"

"One of the most crucial findings in our understanding of menopausal symptoms is how diverse they are," social psychologist Dr. Carol Tavris, coauthor, along with Dr. Avrum Bluming, of *Estrogen Matters*, told me. "No wonder women don't put them together as all part of a menopausal package. You have joint pain and muscle pain, so you go to a rheumatologist. You have heart palpitations, so you go to a cardiologist. You are depressed, so you go to a psychiatrist. When you understand them all as part of the physiological changes of the plummet of estrogen and other aspects of menopause, suddenly the scales fall from your eyes."

There are so many other symptoms people don't realize are menopause related. Heart palpitations are another big one.

Dr. Casperson told me: "So I'm having coffee in the surgeon's lounge, and one of my friends comes in—she's a forty-eight-year-old vascular surgeon, highly educated. She tells me, 'I'm going to the cardiologist. My heart palpitations are so bad, I don't feel safe driving my kids anymore.' Then I saw her again and she said, 'The cardiac workup was negative. They said my heart's totally fine. I still don't feel safe driving.' I said, 'Sounds like perimenopause. You should try some hormones.' So she goes to her doctor, who chooses a medication for her to try. She comes back and says, 'The heart palpitations are completely gone. Why didn't my cardiologist tell me this? They just told me I was fine.' Here's this very capable woman in her forties who was *going to stop driving.*"

I can't get over how often women's discomfort is ignored and how much I've minimized it in my own life. That's why I named my company Stripes Beauty. We've earned our stripes! We deserve to feel our best. No more shrinking. Time to feel good about our cumulative experiences, and unapologetically so.

"With men, no one seems to ask them, 'Are you suffering enough?'" said Dr. Casperson. "Whereas I think women get that question. I say, they had to pay for parking, get childcare, take off work to get into a doctor's office—that's suffering. It's already a lot of work. But we never ask a guy when he comes in with low energy, low testosterone, erectile dysfunction, 'Are you suffering enough with that to justify the treatment?'"

The bottom line: We don't have to suffer at this age; we deserve to feel better . . . even great. I know I've said a lot about how frustrating and lonely it can be trying to find solutions to the problems associated with menopause, so I should also note how good it feels when you finally get it all under control.

Things They Really Should Tell Us About Hot Flashes, UTIs, and Other Discomforts

- To combat hot flashes, wear layers and cotton fabrics. Sleep and stay hydrated. Monitor your triggers.

- Symptoms related to blood vessel dilation and constriction (hot flashes, night sweats, heart palpitations) are most effectively treated with hormone therapy.

- Genitourinary syndrome of menopause is common and often manifests as urine leakage, frequent UTIs, vaginal dryness, or painful intercourse. This syndrome can also be treated by hormone therapy.

- GI issues can be addressed with a healthy diet, probiotics, and hormone therapy.

- While some doctors say to take a small dose of antibiotics preventatively, taking antibiotics for every UTI can create a vicious cycle of GI issues. Consider breaking the cycle with vaginal estrogen.

- Lifestyle changes can make a difference in every area of health. So hydrate, eat well, sleep, manage stress, and exercise. Yes, we are given these instructions all the time, and, yes, they are easier said than done! I'll break them down later in the book and offer realistic help.

CHAPTER TWO

MY INFERTILITY
STORY

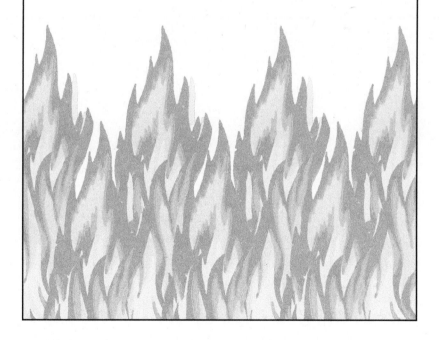

Every woman has a story of how she realized that menopause had come for her. For me, the close-to-menopause news came at the same time as the you-probably-won't-get-naturally-pregnant news. I entered menopause and motherhood at more or less the same time, becoming in one fell swoop both mother and crone. And both struggles—with early menopause and infertility—had me drenched in sweat, confusion, and shame.

I always dreamed I'd be a young mother but never got around to it. Then I found a partner who wanted to be a parent, too. Within three months, Liev and I had made the decision to start a family. I'd spent my entire adult life up to that point trying to avoid pregnancy, and so once I felt ready, at age thirty-six, I assumed I'd get pregnant on my first go—maybe my second or third at most. Months went by. Nothing. When I'd seen the doctor to find out why I wasn't getting pregnant and been told I was nearing menopause, I coursed with shame. *What use am I if I can't bear children? Did I become an old lady without even noticing? How could I have let this happen? What have I done wrong?* I flashed back to every time I'd ever done something I knew was bad for me, every crash diet, being on birth control for fifteen years. *My body doesn't work because I abused it!* I thought. *Of course it won't let me have a baby, because I'm not fit to be a mother!* How does guilt and shame send you into such dark places and to beliefs you would never normally consider? It's almost as if those feelings are the self-sabotaging you think you deserve. When in doubt, blame everything on yourself!

Even though Liev had been nothing but supportive, I was scared to tell him. I was gaslighting myself. I thought, *If he wants a family and I can't have babies, he won't want me anymore.* I felt that when I was told I was close to menopause, I'd been branded an unproductive, barren person. The shame bled into all parts of my life, because I wasn't being completely up front about this perhaps futile pursuit to get pregnant, which was taking up every spare moment and part of my brain.

But I pulled myself together and tried to focus on *not being menopausal*. And as much as possible I avoided talking about it with Liev or anyone else. I enlisted his help when I needed to, but I took it on mostly as my job to figure it out. Deep down, I believed this natural course of events could be altered on my own with enough hard work. I'd had to prove my worth in my career and in finding the right partner. Before those things happened, I'd made it clear how badly I wanted them—so why should my fertility be any different? If it was my fault for ending up in this predicament, then surely I had the power to get myself out.

Yes, I know that's stupid. In retrospect, if a woman said anything like that to me, I'd tell her, "We are much more than our fertility. There are plenty of ways to have a family. If you feel you can't share something like this with your partner, maybe the relationship isn't on a solid footing." But at the time some regressive part of me thought, *Well, isn't fertility part of women's worth? Aren't we here to reproduce?*

I was determined to get pregnant as soon as possible. Because of my hormone levels, I wasn't a candidate for IVF, but I tried fertility drugs like Clomid and procedures like intrauterine insemination (IUI). I would have eaten my dog's toenails if someone told me it would help. I tracked my ovulation and checked my temperature on the regular. I even got scans to see the follicles and the eggs forming, and we'd have sex at the exact optimal moment for conception. None of it worked.

Since this was eighteen years ago, the internet wasn't yet what it is today. I couldn't even find the chat rooms that did exist. Some friends of mine swore by Chinese medicine. I'd tried acupuncture already and some herbal teas. And as luck would have it, about five months into this process I went to shoot a movie in China.

While the rest of the cast were sightseeing or resting on their days off, I was hunting down a top herbalist at a hospital in Beijing. At first I tried to navigate the process on my own—and it was comical attempting to explain to the taxi driver where I wanted to go. I soon realized I would get nowhere fast without a translator, and my lovely young production assistant volunteered to help me. She remained game and professional even as she translated phrases like "shrinking ovaries."

Meanwhile, I sat in horror, my eyes darting from the doctor to the translator as the bad news rolled out before me in two languages. Everyone in the room was at sea: I, with my failing body, struggling to make myself understood; the PA, grappling for obscure gynecologic vocabulary; and the doctor, wondering if my translator was getting it right. *Did I understand that it was very unlikely I'd get pregnant?* Yes, that part I got loud and clear! A firm *no* is a very clear universal language! No need for any charades: I was a failure as a woman!

After having discussed my compromised fertility in great and graphic detail, and with plenty of mortifying hand gestures for sex, the doctor sent me away with a ton of herbs. From that point on, I was brewing teas that would stink up any room I was in. When the movie wrapped, I smuggled giant laundry bags filled with teas back home and drank them every day for months.

Just thinking about those smells makes me gag now. Lots of people around me were saying, "Be careful with that stuff! Some herbs can hurt your liver!" But at the time there was nothing I wouldn't do to have a baby. I didn't care if they weren't FDA approved. "I'll worry about my liver later," I said.

Eventually, an endocrinologist recommended a book called *Inconceivable: A Woman's Triumph over Despair and Statistics* by Julia Indichova. The author had, as I did, an elevated FSH (follicle-stimulating hormone, which stimulates the ovaries to prepare eggs for ovulation and which appears in higher levels in menopausal women). She'd tried everything the doctors had told her to do. Finally, she decided to develop her own program. The book made me feel real hope for the first time since this journey had begun. Sometimes a simple sense of identification can be the beginning of healing. I started my own intuitive plan. I went on a very strict anti-inflammatory diet. I churned up wefts of wheatgrass every day. I began to feel that I lived in the produce section of Whole Foods.

I was peeing on sticks constantly, both to track my ovulation and to check for pregnancy if my period was even an hour late. I was monitoring the pH of my vagina because I'd heard that sperm do better in an alkaline environment than an acidic one. I spent so much money, but I would have mortgaged my house to try to solve this problem. I became disheartened by the whole fertility process. I began looking into adoption, and I researched donor eggs as well. There was a brief moment when I thought my partner's sperm might have been to blame, but nope, the tests showed *he* was fine. Then I had one pregnancy. I thought, *This is it! I turned back the tide! I did the impossible!*

Less than two months later, I miscarried.

I was back to the starting point again. I'd come to learn that, according to the Mayo Clinic, at age thirty-five, the miscarriage risk is about one in five; at age forty the risk is 33 to 40 percent. At age forty-five, it's 57 to 80 percent.

Another few months went by, and nothing. The sperm and the egg were still not working together. And by this point, as a couple, we were losing steam. My obsession created a strain on our relationship. I was driving myself crazy, and the derangement was spreading. We were at the brink of giving up on a pregnancy and maybe each other.

What's more, I was still struggling with shame about infertility—I kept the book *Inconceivable* hidden under my mattress. I was perplexed by how ill-prepared I was for my new perimenopausal reality. How confusing it could be! One article I've since read about perimenopause described period durations month to month as having all the regularity of a locker combination—more likely to be 29-45-17 than 28-28-28.

Why had my doctors not found it important to help set me up for this thing that was always coming? Periods start. Then they stop. Period! It's all part of the plan. It was always how it was supposed to go. It's not a failing. Why is it shrouded in secrecy? And even when you own up to it, why is it so damn confusing?

One younger friend of mine learned that she was nearing early menopause only when she went in to freeze her eggs. She took a useful blood test that tracked her anti-Mullerian hormone level. The AMH test doesn't tell you how fertile you are, but it gives you a sense of how many eggs you have left. So a typical number for a twenty-five-year-old might be 3.0 nanograms per milliliter, and for a forty-five-year-old it's more likely to be something like 0.5. When the number is zero, you're in menopause. Her starting number, at age thirty-four, was 0.3. And so she wound up on a years-long run of trying every fertility treatment in the book.

"Because my body took forever to recruit follicles, I often exceeded the 'safe' dosage of a drug," she said. "For example, I can never take Clomid again because I took so much of it that I started having vision problems! At some of these fertility clinics it's like this 'anything for the eggs!' attitude, like the rest of your physical and mental health is just collateral damage."

She'd been on birth control since age sixteen, then went immediately into the IVF process. "I was taking drugs off-label and not knowing which way was up. Then I started to have crazy hot flashes, night sweats, and depression."

After years of trying countless treatments, her body was able to generate one egg that was successfully fertilized. It's now frozen and waiting to be implanted. She was hoping to get lucky before inseminating it, but her doctor told her: "You're past IVF now, but we can monitor you constantly to see if your body has any last spurts of ovulation. Then we'll try to catch that ovulation into an IUI. But we've tried that three times over the past year. None of them has been successful."

And so she's left with this one embryo. At the age of thirty-eight, it's probably her last shot. The process has taken such a toll on her body and her mental health. What she's describing has been called "disenfranchised grief," mourning the loss of a potential future and doing it alone: "My relationship to my body, to my reproductive organs is completely changed because of the constant invasive procedures. Just how many more vaginal ultrasounds can I freaking get?"

I find this story so heartbreaking, emblematic of the tightrope so many women walk and the hard work and focus it takes to move through the shame and vulnerability.

My friend Mary Coustas, author of *All I Know: A Memoir of Love, Loss, and Life,* did seventeen rounds of IVF over a period of ten years. She gave birth to her only child at the age of fifty-one.

In the midst of my own crisis over the toll fertility treatments were taking on me, I left to shoot the thriller *Eastern Promises* in London. A few weeks into the filming, I began to feel strange, and I went to a pharmacy—I can still picture it—and bought a British pregnancy test. In my rented house, I stared at the test and saw the faintest line appear. Then slowly it got stronger, until it was a full, clear, solid line. Undeniable. The line was yelling at me: "I'm here!"

I called Liev and told him.

"Wow! Well, let's see," he said. He sounded thrilled but cautious, and I was beside myself with joy, though also afraid I'd lose this pregnancy, too. It didn't help that I had to ride a three-hundred-pound Russian motorbike for that movie. The director, David Cronenberg, adored motorbikes and was enthusiastic about me being the real rider. I'd ridden a Vespa before, but this was a monster compared to that. I was up for the challenge. It was nothing compared to some of the other risky things I'd done in the past. For a photoshoot to promote *King Kong,* I had to stand on the top of the Chrysler Building so that the Empire State Building was visible in the background. In that case, my manager looked at the harness I was supposed to climb into and said, "You don't have to do this. It seems insane." I was afraid of heights.

But my assistant said, "I'd do it," and my competitive streak got the better of me. I took off my high heels and climbed barefoot onto the gargoyle. I let them do one roll of film as the wind whipped around me before I said I thought that was probably enough of that. And back then I hadn't been pregnant.

After three or four motorbike lessons, I could ride around with seeming confidence, then park in front of the camera, take my helmet off, and shake out my hair. I tried to make it look effortless, but meanwhile, all that was running through my head during those scenes were terrified thoughts: *Oh my God, this is so dangerous! I don't want to lose this baby! I cannot lose this baby!*

I also didn't want to tell anyone yet, because it was so early, and because I didn't want to be difficult, so I just kept going. It was yet another example of how as women we often do things that put us at risk in order to be team players. Once I'd convinced everyone that I could ride the motorbike, they gave me more riding to do. There was one scene in which I had to ride the thing at night with Viggo Mortensen on the back, and in film they always wet down the roads to make it look better. I was so scared. I had a baby inside me and a fully grown adult on the back of the bike with no helmet. But I did it, and then I went back to my rented house, shaking and full of gratitude that I'd made it through another day.

A few weeks later, while I was doing a scene with Sinéad Cusack, I felt the first flutter. It was a sensation I'd never had in my life, but I knew instantly what it meant: the baby was moving around. The baby was real. The baby was fighting and strong. My eyes welled with tears. The scene was not sad. Crying made no sense in that moment, so it was good that the camera was focused on Sinéad. She stayed professional and made it through as if nothing was amiss. But after the take she said, "What happened? Are you okay?"

I leaned over and whispered to her, "I'm pregnant, and I think I just felt the baby move for the first time." Then I burst into tears.

"Oh God, love, love, love!" she said, cooing over me and holding me while I wept.

I'm sure everyone on the set was baffled, but we stood like that for a long time.

I had two thoughts while she soothed me: One: *I will always love this woman for being kind to me in this moment.* Two: *I'm not riding that fucking motorbike anymore.*

I gave birth at thirty-eight, and I had my second baby very soon after, when I was forty. I guess my body had somehow learned the program to make babies. I was still breastfeeding when I got pregnant the second time, but the baby had teeth and was biting, so I was supplementing as well to give my breasts time to heal. I always knew I wanted more than one baby, though I didn't expect it to happen so soon. I'd wanted more than two, actually—but alas, by that point time really had run out.

Several doctors told me women past forty can, theoretically, still get pregnant naturally, and they might not know when they're in a fertile window, because they might ovulate sporadically. If you're having irregular cycles and seeing menopause-range numbers when you have your hormones tested, you could be in perimenopause, which can go on for even longer than a decade.

Dr. Sharon Malone warned: "Just because you're in perimenopause, it doesn't mean you can't get pregnant. It's less likely that you will conceive, however a higher percentage of the pregnancies in perimenopausal women are unplanned—simply because they think they can't get pregnant." A friend of mine found this out when she had a "surprise" baby in her forties, after her older two were nearing the end of elementary school. The baby was a joy, but it disrupted her plans to go back to school, and she said more than once she'd been asked on the playground if she was the baby's grandmother.

(Yes, this goes on the list with questions like "Are you pregnant?" that should never, ever, be asked, because heaven help you if the answer is no. I have a friend who had the best response to someone who asked her this: "Unless you see the baby crowning, never ask a woman this.")

Dr. Jen Gunter, author of *The Vagina Bible* and *The Menopause Manifesto,* became more aware of the need for doctors to bring patients into the process when she faced issues in her own pregnancy.

"My children were born very prematurely, at twenty-six weeks, and had a lot of health problems," she told me. "I appreciated the importance of having good information. I started to realize that there's this massive communication gap in medicine. It's like how I feel when someone talks about computers. My brain stops working. There are all kinds of gaps in medicine and people seeking to exploit those gaps, and I'm just trying to fill them with real information."

When it comes to pregnancy in middle age, she said, "Pregnancy at this age is one of those low-probability, very high-consequence things. Would this be a good thing for you or not a good thing? And if it could be a good thing for you, are you aware of the much higher risk of chromosomal abnormalities? What would that mean for you?"

The frustrations of perimenopause aren't limited to women trying to get pregnant. Dr. Suzanne Gilberg-Lenz, the legendary ob-gyn of Beverly Hills and author of *Menopause Bootcamp,* told me the worst part of perimenopause is "the ups and the downs that people are having when their hormones are fluctuating, and they can't predict how they're going to feel on any given day. I think when we arrange so much of our lives around our periods, we identify with them. It seems like we're always supposed to somehow manage our cycle, trying to get pregnant or not get pregnant.

"That's decades of our lives. And we start to think that's who we are: *Oh, that week's not going to be a good week for a decision or activity, or I'm going on vacation. How can I not have my period the whole time?* We orient ourselves around this one physiologic aspect that can feel dominant. So I think that people can feel very confused about who they are when cycling becomes irregular or stops. We spend a lot of life preparing for menstruation, being in it, recovering from it. Then when our cycle is gone, we realize we'd psychologically and physiologically been living with this biologic partner all those years. You don't expect your period to become a hole in your life, but then it does."

I found this really rang true to me. Being fertile women, as we're reminded each month by our periods, we can become wrapped up in fertility being part of our identity. When our periods are suddenly gone, we question who we are and if we are suddenly whole new people. The world might see you differently, and you might see yourself differently, too. You might ask big, panicky questions like *Who am I now? Will I ever get myself back?* Or even darker ones, like *Am I invisible now? Is this the end?*

"As in any grieving process, I think we have to give ourselves grace," Dr. Gilberg-Lenz told me. "I hit menopause recently, when my daughter turned twenty-three. And I'm going to tell you, I immediately felt better. I said, 'Okay, so this is how dudes are? It's great!' I'm so much chiller now that I don't have erratic cycles and surprise periods."

One vibrant friend told me that based on what she'd heard, she figured she'd enter menopause in her fifties. Then at age forty-two she was at her ob-gyn for an annual exam, and the doctor said during an ultrasound, "I can't find your ovaries because they're so tiny and shrunken. I'm surprised you're even still bleeding. You are approaching the end of the menopause season."

Like me, she was completely shocked: "I had no idea. I wish that someone had told me that when I was thirty-nine, the year that every single part of my body became unfamiliar to me—my digestive system, my skin, my hair, my emotions. It felt like a different body that I had to get used to. And I look back now and I see that was perimenopause. Had I had the language for that, I could have started hormones, or at least known that I wasn't sick; it wasn't a disease. It also wasn't a mental health issue. It was this natural process."

She mourned all the lost years of pleasure she might have had with better education. "Had that been even on the radar, I could have taken better care of myself. The advice that I would give to anybody is: If you're feeling out of control of what's happening in your body, get to the doctor quickly, advocate for yourself, and ask for help. Read about it. Learn about it. I did everything late and I was always playing catch-up. I could have addressed each symptom more effectively. Instead, I was screwed up for several years."

We need to be reminded that we should be compassionate with ourselves. None of the choices we have to make are easy. So many of us spend time up to our forties wondering, *Am I going to have children? Am I not? If I do, how am I going to handle it? Am I going to be a good mom? Am I going to be a bad one? What will happen with my career if I take time off for caregiving? Am I a bad mom if I go back to work right away?* And after we've gone through menopause, we get closer to making decisions based entirely on what we want to do, not what others want from us. This is the age when we realize that all through our lives, we've felt pressured by and succumbed to expectations and hormones that we didn't necessarily sign up for.

Lately I've been having a lot of powerful conversations with women about the complicated feelings we've had about no longer being able to become pregnant. One friend of mine recently got an IUD at the age of forty-eight to help her deal with heavy and irregular periods. "I couldn't believe how much it hurt getting it put in," she told me after the appointment. "Why don't they warn you? I started sobbing on the table. I was already emotional because I was thinking of it as the official end of my fertility—by the time it comes out I will likely be in full menopause and there will be no chance of another pregnancy. It made me sad to say goodbye to that period of my life, especially in such a painful way, even if it was on my own terms."

A couple of weeks later, after the cramps from the insertion had stopped and she'd had some more time to think, she felt better about the decision and that time of her life: "My therapist said, 'Don't ever use the phrase 'end of my fertility' again! Fertility is much bigger than being able to get pregnant and give birth. It's time now to think about what fertility means to you at this point in your life. Is it writing? Is it making art? Is it taking care of other people's children? Is it being a good friend? No one is taking care of the earth and the people on it except for us. That's fertility, too."

Things They Really Should Tell Us About Fertility

- Periods change a lot during perimenopause. They can become much lighter or heavier and more or less frequent.

- The chance of getting pregnant declines over time. If you're over age thirty-five and want to conceive but haven't naturally in six months of trying, consult a fertility specialist. Get ready for the term "geriatric pregnancy"!

- The rate of miscarriage rises with age. At age thirty-five, it's about one in five; at age forty, 33 to 40 percent; at age forty-five, it's 57 to 80 percent.

- Until it's been a full year since you've had a period, pregnancy is still possible. If you're up for the challenges of having a baby late in life, Godspeed. But if you're sure you don't want to get pregnant, talk to your ob-gyn about birth control options.

- There's way more to fertility than being able to bear a child.

CHAPTER THREE

VAG OF HONOR

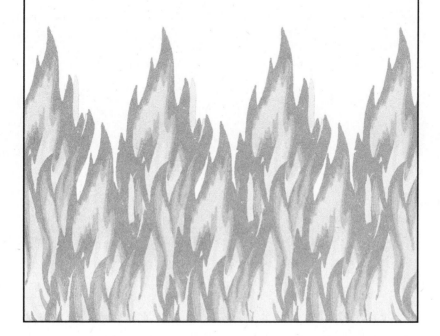

L et's face it—sex is an issue in middle age. Many women give up on it altogether. Those of us trying to stay in the game face untold indignities and surprises. Personally, I found myself in the situation of being a menopausal woman when I started dating again after many years of being in a relationship, and I confess that when it came to matters of attraction and then of logistics, I didn't quite know what I was doing.

I met Billy not long after my breakup, though by that point I had been separated for a year. I didn't know for the longest time that my costar on a TV show was going to be the person I belonged with. There were no signals going off. I was in no mood for romance or flirting. I planned to hold myself together for my kids and keep my head down at work. Like so many women my age, I found my libido wasn't what it had been in my twenties. Maybe one day I'd find love again, but I knew I wouldn't be looking for it for the foreseeable future—and certainly not at work.

Interestingly, *Gypsy*, the show I was on at the time, had me, in my late forties, playing the most sexual role of my career, a horny, sociopathic therapist. Billy and I chatted on set during lighting changes, and I'd have said we were friendly. But for a very long time, that was as far as it went. I was so closed off to love that in the months and months of shooting, even after we'd simulated sex onscreen many times, dry-humping each other to the point of exhaustion, I hadn't given romance with him a thought.

Then one day during a sex scene, he spontaneously flung a pillow across the room while ravishing me with such passion that I blushed and broke character: *Oh! Why, hello, sailor!* I thought to myself as me, not as the woman I was playing. Then: *Wait, that felt like . . . something.*

Soon after, during one of those lengthy lighting changes, while we were having a meaningful conversation, we exchanged a look.

It was held just a beat too long to be anything other than shared attraction. We also had mutual friends trying to matchmake, and we started flirting via text. Before long, our feelings were undeniable: we were falling in love.

When he and I were finally about to sleep together off camera, I politely excused myself before things got hot and frisky, as if I were saying, "Let me slip into something more comfortable . . . I'll be right back." Like it was 1953 and I had a negligee in my purse. Then I went into the bathroom before getting naked and furiously attempted to scratch a hormone patch off my body.

I'd started wearing the patch a couple of years earlier for hormone therapy. I was worried that if he saw it he would realize it meant I was menopausal: no longer a vibrant, fertile being. What if he wanted another child?

Unfortunately, the patch's adhesive leaves a mark on the skin that's very hard to get rid of. The doctor had said, "To take it off, just get car oil from the hardware store." When I told him I didn't want to pour car oil on my body, he shrugged and said, "Well, it's the only thing that works." Since then, people have recommended baby oil, coconut oil, nail polish remover, eye makeup remover, loofahs, rubbing alcohol, and medical adhesive remover to me. Every strategy has its camp of supporters. Most women I know just scrub it off in the shower using shower gel or an oil-based cleanser with a washcloth.

Having told him to hold on for just a minute, I ripped it off and scrubbed the skin raw.

"Is everything okay in there?" he called, because I was taking so long.

I came out mortified.

"What's wrong?" he asked.

I stumbled and reached for words, but nothing would quite come out.

"Are you okay?" he said, with a gentle hand on my arm.

"Menopause!" I blurted out. "I didn't want to tell you."

Suddenly the words came gushing out. "I wear these hormone

patches, and I didn't want you to see it because then you would know I'm in early menopause, which means I am *old*, and you wouldn't want me and, *Oh my God, should I just leave?*"

A smile broke over his face. He seemed very relieved that the issue wasn't a lack of desire.

Phew.

He told me he thought it was great I was taking care of myself, and he asked me how he could help.

Double phew.

He added that he could hardly be surprised; we were the same age, after all: "Hey, if it makes you feel better: I've got gray hairs on my balls."

Swoon.

Oh my God! Reader, that *did* make me feel better. Those to date remain the most romantic words I've ever heard, onscreen or off, and that includes the script of every movie I've ever been in, and even this same man's very loving marriage proposal, which came seven years later.

We were in it together, this aging thing. I knew then that we could help each other deal with whatever happened. Shame I'd been carrying for years went away in that moment. I was able to share with him honestly what I was experiencing even though it didn't match with what I thought was appropriate for a sexy new girlfriend. He was compassionate, not squeamish or awkward. That was a great gift. My hormone patches never got in the way of sex again.

It's exhausting holding secrets and such a waste of time. As soon as I'd spilled the beans on menopause with Billy, and upon receiving his great response, I started talking about it more with my friends, and when I stopped hiding what was going on, I found myself more confident than I'd ever been before.

There are enough things to make us feel bad in this life—I swear, my "smart home" is out to destroy me—so we shouldn't invent new ones. What a waste, fighting to feel and look younger than I was. (Though it's no surprise that I'd internalized those messages about holding on to youth at all costs: remember when Anne Bancroft played the ancient Mrs. Robinson to Dustin Hoffman's graduate, even though he was only *six years* younger than she was?) There are still plenty of vestiges of the archaic belief in women's "unfuckability" beyond a certain age—this, in spite of so many powerful figures I admired when I was coming up in the business, like Rene Russo, Angela Bassett, Kim Basinger, Grace Jones, Susan Sarandon, Jessica Lange. They were and still are sex on legs!

I'm always eager to see more storytelling about women getting what they want rather than narratives built around women as the objects of that desire.

While many of us find our libido plummeting in middle age, some people find themselves able to embrace a new form of sexuality that feels good for them, because they know themselves, and they lose the awkwardness of youth. There is, though, often a fear of change or a period of adjustment before we find our desire again.

For me it's reassuring that all the doctors I've spoken with have told me a changing libido is completely normal and that there are things we can do about it if we want to.

"It is quite common that women will experience a decrease in libido during the menopausal transition," Dr. Sharon Malone told me. "And it's no surprise if you are tired, if you're having hot flashes, if you haven't had a good night's sleep, you're irritable and you feel bad generally that you don't want to have sex. And did I mention your vagina's dry, and sex is painful? Duh, you're not in the mood. When you don't feel well, you don't want sex. Who wants to have sex after they haven't slept in three months?"

Friends of mine say there are strong psychological and relational components affecting when they want to have sex. One said, "How can you be a partner in the bedroom when you just brought home spicy Dijon and I asked for yellow mustard? Get your shit together."

Menopause affects couples in all sorts of ways. I asked my most macho friend (who served in the Marines) about his experience of menopause. He said, "My girl sweats all over me all night, and I have seen her literally shaving her face! I still wanna have sex with her! I think it's totally unfair that women have to go through this. Childbirth is hard enough . . . and now *this*?! Come on! Men have it so easy compared to women. It's another round of women showing extreme strength, but it breaks my heart to see my wife suffer."

From some partners of the menopausal women with whom I've spoken, I hear things like "I didn't know my wife anymore." Or "I didn't know why she no longer wanted to have sex with me." Or "Why is she always mad at me?"

One lesbian couple I know was thrown into crisis when one of the partners, who was ten years older, went into menopause and lost her libido. The younger partner said she hadn't signed up for a sexless relationship, so if her wife wasn't going to do anything about improving their sex life, she'd like to transition to an open marriage and start dating other people.

And yet, some women find themselves feeling very sexual as they enter menopause.

"Sometimes the hormonal fluctuations in perimenopause can increase sexual desire," Dr. Malone said. (Some women experience surges of estrogen and testosterone that leave them more turned on than ever.) "Those women may say, 'I've never felt more sexual in my life than in my forties.' If that's happening for you, great! And while that may be true for some, that's not the lived experience of most women."

One doctor working to improve sexual lives in menopause is Dr. Somi Javaid, the founder of HerMD and an expert in hypoactive sexual desire disorder (HSDD). She told me that before we can understand sex during menopause, we have to understand female sexuality itself: "A lot of times, for men, sexuality is like an on-and-off switch. With women, when you talk about sexuality, you have to talk about the biopsychosocial approach: relationships, hormones, what's going on in their lives, other medical concerns."

For example: many women in middle age start to struggle with bladder control, because with the decline of estrogen, there's a decline in the bladder's elasticity and muscle strength. This can complicate our desire to be intimate with others. So many friends have been telling me they have to make much more effort now to keep it all together when they laugh or cough, and they're wondering if they should try pelvic floor therapy—which might involve stretching, tailored exercises like Kegels, or electrical stimulation to relax the pelvic floor muscles. (I've been told it's good to do three sets of ten Kegel contractions a day, and that if you're trying to find the right muscles, imagine you stop peeing midstream. When I'm bored enough, I remember to do them. Dear reader, I hope you're not doing them now! Actually, let's pause here and do a round together.)

Thank goodness there are doctors taking women's sexual experience seriously. I asked Dr. Stacy Lindau, professor at the University of Chicago and director of the Program in Integrative Sexual Medicine (PRISM), what is the one thing all of us could benefit from knowing about, and she introduced me to the bulbocavernosus muscle. "This muscle is the most important muscle in a woman's body that nobody's ever heard of," she said.

"The bulbocavernosus muscle is around the opening to the vagina, and it talks to the brain. So when the muscle's not causing a problem, it's just there, and when we want it to open, we can consciously open it by bearing down a little bit. Those of us who've given birth vaginally know about bearing down to open this muscle. The physiology of sexual arousal naturally sends signals to this muscle to tell it to be receptive to sexual penetration. But sometimes even with the physiology sending the messages, if there's been pain before, the brain is telling the muscle, 'Don't open! It's not safe! It's going to hurt!'"

In other words, the brain will keep the vaginal sphincter from opening, and then if you try to have sex anyway, it will hurt, and then the vagina will close up even more. Combine that with vaginal dryness, and no wonder libido tends to go down in middle age. Dr. Lindau went on, "Many women will say something to me like 'I feel like I'm a virgin again. It's so painful.' Or they'll say, 'It feels like his penis is hitting a wall.' And what does a woman think if she never had that problem before and now it feels like the penis is hitting up against something in the vagina? She will say, 'Do I have cancer, a tumor that's blocking the penis from going in?'

"Never once have I seen a tumor as the answer to the question. The explanation almost always is an involuntary spasm of the bulbocavernosus muscle. The penis is hitting this wall of muscle."

What can be done about it? Lots, as it turns out! "Sometimes teaching women about this muscle and giving them the bearing-down suggestion is really helpful. We often add some lubricant for sex and some moisturizer for daily use or prescribe estrogen if she can do that. Other times we can use self-dilation with graduated vaginal dilators or pelvic floor physical therapy or all of the above."

And this is how I came to google "vaginal dilators" at my desk on a Tuesday afternoon. Mercifully, I'm not finding a link that suggests the lower drawer in your refrigerator for cucumbers and carrots. In fact, they're a bunch of upright phalluses in cheery rainbow colors. Often in flexible silicone, vaginal dilators range in size from small all the way up to the size of a terrifyingly large penis. Dr. Lindau said, "Self-dilation can be accomplished by starting with a dilator size that's small enough to easily be inserted by a woman into her vagina, then doing some exercises with that to build confidence and capacity and then progressing to the next size, and then the next. And usually people's goal would be to be able to accommodate a vaginal dilator that's a little bit bigger than their partner's erect penis or whatever toy or dildo they want to use."

More or less the opposite problem, vaginal prolapse, where the top of the vagina sags into the vaginal canal, also has various fixes, from surgical repair to pelvic floor therapy.

Another therapy tool that looks like a Fisher-Price toy is the stackable penis ring (one brand is Ohnut). When someone is experiencing deep pain (which should of course be checked out by a doctor!), Dr. Javaid encourages patients to explore buffer rings to be used with sexual health tools or a penis, depending on the sexual partner. This allows the patient to determine the depth of penetration to reduce pain while still providing sensation.

Dr. Kelly Casperson told me that many vaginal symptoms can be traced to low estrogen, so she encourages women to explore hormone therapy or an estrogen cream prescribed by a doctor and applied to the vagina. She adds that if you don't have a doctor who will talk to you about symptom relief, find a new doctor. And don't feel bad about whatever helps you: "When people say, 'I don't want to use lube or a vibrator,' I say, 'I have two vibrators for my mouth, an electric toothbrush and a water flosser. Why can't I have a vibrator down there, too?"

I agree! I was given a vibrator by a friend at my bachelorette party—it's shaped like a rose, glows in the dark, and has multiple speeds—and let me tell you, it is *excellent*. Similarly, there should be no shame in reading erotica or looking at pornography if it aids your libido. Doctors told me that a lot of women think finding ways to get in the mood for a partner on our own is cheating, but it's really just signaling the body to prepare for sex, which means encouraging physical and emotional arousal.

And why should we deny ourselves pleasure? One night I was in the mood but on my own, so when I got out of a bath I got into bed with my brand-new rose vibrator. I realized that it had a sucking feature, so I decided to try that out on my nipple. I know it's not common to engage in foreplay with yourself—usually you just get straight to the deed. But for this particular night, I decided I would take my time with myself. Well, it all went well. Afterward, I put the rose back in the box, and then I left it beside me, like we were going to have postcoital pillow talk. The next morning, my fifteen-year-old came in and saw the box and said, "Mom!"

"All women have vibrators!" I said. "You can get them at Urban Outfitters now!"

But I was mortified. And on top of that, my nipple was throbbing *all day*. Maybe I need to read the full instructions on the various functions. Fine print has never been my strong suit.

The point is, if you're sexually unhappy, it's not true that there's nothing you can do about it except make yourself try to have intercourse more. This is the "use it or lose it" fallacy.

"There is a rumor that women should have sex to prevent what used to be called 'vaginal atrophy,' and was called something even worse in the 1980s: 'senile vagina,'" Dr. Casperson told me. "The truth is that atrophy comes from your hormone levels going down, not from putting something in your vagina or not. The rumor comes from an ob-gyn paper looking at women who came in who were sexually active, and women who came in who were not sexually active. The sexually active women had less atrophy. And from that, the study's authors concluded that sex prevents atrophy. But that's not what that study shows. It shows that people with less atrophy stayed more sexually active—I'm guessing because sex wasn't painful for them. To tell women that they should have sex to prevent a hormonal change drives me insane."

Quick sidebar: Why is the male term "erectile dysfunction" so much more palatable? "Erectile dysfunction" sounds like an issue with your dishwasher that a handyman could fix in fifteen minutes. "Vaginal atrophy" sounds like *doom*. Again: don't get me started on doctors telling pregnant women in their midthirties that they are having a *geriatric pregnancy*.

Dr. Casperson said hormone therapy can work wonders on atrophy, or whatever you call it, as can lifestyle changes: "Stress is also horrible on the sex drive. Sleep is important. 'Exhausted' is not good for sex drive. We have data on shift workers. They have much lower libido and interest in sex because their sleep-wake cycles are messed up. Communication is so important."

Here are some of the questions she encourages us to ask: Why do we want to have sex? Why do we want to continue to be intimate? What does sex mean to us? How can we prioritize it? What feels good? These are particularly good questions to ask in the context of couples counseling or with the help of a sex therapist.

Pelvic-floor issues are just one aspect of female health that can affect sexual desire or pleasure. A woman may have unresolved trauma that causes her to shut down in sexual situations, a negative body image, or medication side effects.

When I asked Dr. Javaid to identify the biggest misconception she sees in her practice, she said it's that there are no options for menopausal sexual health. Women may even have heard this from a medical practitioner, which is likely, because only about 30 percent of ob-gyns are trained in menopause.

There are two FDA-approved medications for women's low sex drive that are often covered by insurance and that I have yet to try. One is a little pink nonhormonal pill called Addyi, which after a couple of weeks can increase excitation and decrease inhibition. The second, Vyleesi, is an injectable (you give yourself a shot in the abdomen or thigh). It works on a different set of neurotransmitters, and it's on demand (like Viagra), so you take it about forty-five minutes before you're planning to have sex.

A doctor investigating your sexual health might administer a questionnaire called the Female Sexual Function Index, which measures libido, orgasm, arousal, pain, satisfaction, and lubrication. (If you're anything like me and you loved the days of doing the quizzes in *Cosmopolitan*, you might actually enjoy it. You can find the quiz online.) Doctors say that a woman who comes in complaining about sexual problems might have an issue in just one of these areas or in all six. And there are different solutions for each of the realms of concern.

One potential sexual-health therapy you may have heard about is testosterone. You might be thinking, *Isn't that a male hormone?* In 2019, the International Menopause Society came out with a global consensus statement supporting testosterone use in women. Though as of this writing testosterone therapy is still not FDA approved for menopausal women, the Menopause Society said that a testosterone patch providing 300 milligrams per day, or a cream releasing 10 milligrams per day, used with or without estrogen and progestogen therapy, could improve "the frequency of satisfying sexual events, arousal, orgasm, pleasure, responsiveness, and self-image."

Women sometimes say they're afraid that if they take testosterone, they'll develop "male" characteristics. In fact, women naturally have testosterone, though at lower levels than men do; taking testosterone supplements may cause a woman to develop acne or more facial hair, but at these low levels there's unlikely to be anything more extreme, like voice deepening. I've heard that a lot of women find that it boosts libido and energy levels.

I do have one friend who has an extreme horror story about mixing up her dosage. Here's what she told me:

I'd started gaining a lot of weight that I could not get off, so I went to my gynecologist. I'd talked to a few girlfriends who said they were taking testosterone and that it had been really helpful to their diet and exercise routines. They swore it had helped them get rid of belly fat.

When I picked up the box that was prescribed to me, I didn't get counseling from the pharmacist, and I just looked up online how to take it. It seemed that I was supposed to rub some on the backs of both thighs every day. That seemed like a lot. The kind my friends had was just a small amount on the backs of their calves. But I decided to just go with it.

Soon, I began to feel really strange. I started having what I can only describe as episodes of a sort of blind rage, and it was all directed at my husband. I started making stories up about my having affairs. I don't actually remember that much about those months, but apparently from November through January I was crazy to the point that it almost cost me my marriage. My hair also began to fall out, and I began to gain even more weight.

Finally, I sent a message to my general practitioner and said I was gaining weight and wanted to come in for blood work. When I went in, he sat me down and said, "What have you been doing different lately?"

I said, "Well, I'm on an estrogen patch, and a few months ago I started taking testosterone. And lately I've been saying crazy things to my husband and I'm really angry."

"How much testosterone are you taking?" he said.

I told him, and his eyes basically popped out of his head. The thirty tubes my ob-gyn had given me should have lasted 270 days. I'd used them up in twenty-seven.

"Oh no," he said. "You are overdosing, and it's making you psychotic!"

I realize how absurd it was that I was worried about my weight and not about the fact that I was *completely psychotic.*

I didn't go back to see my ob-gyn, but I messaged her, and I just said, "When I wrote and told you I was having an adverse reaction to this medication, you never even inquired as to what that was like."

She later told me she assumed I was having issues with my hair. She had never talked about this possible rage situation. And I felt like she'd given me no guidance in the process. I'm so glad I caught the problem before I fully lost my mind and my marriage, but I'm still never getting those weeks back!

It's important to know that a doctor can help determine the dosage of testosterone for maximum benefit without serious side effects. When I first tried it, I felt flushed and a bit edgy all the time without enough of an upside to make it feel worth my while. I probably could have worked to find the right dosage, but I just opted to stop taking it.

However, on my most recent visit, my gynecologist convinced me to give it another go, and this time I've been really enjoying it. Maybe the dosage is right now or maybe I just didn't need it until now. The lesson I took away is not to rule something out forever just because it didn't work once ten years ago. Menopause is a journey. Circumstances and bodies change, and products evolve—and at least I wasn't taking ten times my recommended dosage!

"No one knows your body better than you do," Dr. Javaid said, encouraging us to trust our instincts about our own health and to find partners who are open to communication about these issues. Sexuality is complicated!

One friend described to me how when she tried to have sex she felt as if "100 knives are piercing my vagina."

"If you give a woman medication to take care of her desire but she's still having pain with intercourse, she's still not going to have sex," Dr. Javaid said when I brought up this problem. "If there's an issue in the relationship where the partner has felt rejected and is now angry and acting out, then even if you ramp up her desire, if you don't fix what's happened in the relationship, the patient is going to 'fail' on a medication that increases libido. It's not really failing. It's that you didn't offer her the full paradigm of care that she needed."

Even premenopause, many women don't want sex unless they feel emotionally close with their partners at the time, whereas men tend to feel close after they've had sex. So this can create a loop of withholding or avoidance. When you throw physiological issues into the mix, this difference can become an insurmountable problem unless you have some difficult adult conversations. That can mean baring your soul, telling hard truths, and being honest about your body's lack of supposed perfection. Done right, all these things can be the hottest form of foreplay. Saying what you want and need tends, I've found, to get everyone way closer to what they want and need way quicker.

Certainly we need to ignore cultural messages that say there's a right or wrong way to do anything, or that we're deficient if we're not like women on TV shows or in porn who have an orgasm from nothing more than a few minutes of penetration, with no lube, conversation, or foreplay. The truth is that fewer than 30 percent of women orgasm just from penetrative intercourse, and even with whatever stimulation we prefer, it takes us, on average, four to ten minutes to have an orgasm on our own, and ten to twenty minutes with a partner.

Men also typically have sexual issues at this time of life. "The body of a man who's in middle age is changing, too," said Dr. Kelly Casperson. "His erection's not going to be as great as it was when he was twenty-three. And some positions don't work as well. And how do we navigate that, so we can still be intimate?" Men in middle age aren't always getting the most thorough medical care themselves, which can affect their female partners. Many experts I spoke with said that men might be told to take Viagra without being asked a single question.

Dr. Casperson told me, "When men come to me for Viagra, I say, 'Have you talked to your partner? Is she interested? Has she seen a doctor? Is she on vaginal estrogen?' Nine times out of ten, they say, 'I haven't talked to her about it.' To which I say, 'So you're in my office, wanting Viagra to put your penis in another person and you didn't talk to the person about that? Where is this penis going to go?'"

I can't count how many women I've heard say they wished their partners had talked with them before taking Viagra. If a woman doesn't have lube and isn't getting the emotional and physical foreplay she needs, it will not be good news that the man in her life can suddenly go all night!

Fortunately, help is available for pretty much any sexual situation you might be facing in menopause. Friends of mine have found their sex drive again after menopause through many different means, including lifestyle changes, hormone therapy, porn, and vibrators. There is no shame in getting help, and there should be no machismo (femachismo?) telling us to "tough it out."

"My mom told me to have a natural birth because she did," Dr. Casperson said. "I'd gone through medical school at this point. I said, 'Mom, we give people pain meds when they break their femur. I'm pretty sure I'm going to take pain meds when I have a baby. Seems like an equal amount of pain. You're wearing shoes, and you drove a car, and you have air-conditioning. Why are you only going natural with your vagina? It makes no sense."

Vibrators, vaginal estrogen, better communication, libido drugs—all of these can contribute to a richer experience of sexuality in middle age. Sex can and should be fun. One friend of mine, when she went from fertile to menopausal, said she was "closed for business, open for pleasure!"

Dr. Emily Morse, host of the podcast *Sex with Emily* and author of *Smart Sex*, told me she faked orgasms until she was thirty-five. She said that in her middle age she finally identified what gave her pleasure and realized that she was spending only 3 percent of her time doing those things. She said, "Pleasure is productive" and "Pleasure begets pleasure." (On that note, please, ladies, can we all start giving our middle-aged friends vibrators as birthday gifts?)

Though of course it's also completely fine to opt out! I have some friends who are just *done* with sex, and more power to them. My mother always said of getting older, "You go to the garden phase of life, whereby you love to watch things grow over time." (To which I always thought, *Uh, I live in a city. There are no gardens near me. And while I love flowers and plants, I have two kids and a dog and some amphibians that require crickets and worms. I'm not equipped to take care of any more living things right now.* Personally, I'd rather sort things out in the bedroom.)

There's no obligation to be sexual or sexy at this or any age. I know women who have happily repurposed that energy for their work or their friendships. And there are plenty of healthy relationships that are nourished by all sorts of intimacy. One friend said, "We cuddle and watch movies, and that's how we stay close." Another: "If I never have sex again, that's fine with me. I just have other priorities now."

Meanwhile, Liz, another friend of mine, is seventy years old and having the best sex of her life.

Like me, Liz didn't get a lot of information from her mother. "My mother couldn't believe how everyone complained about getting older," she told me. "She would say, 'Shall we just all move on? Yes, I'm going through menopause—so, what book are you reading?'"

That made Liz think that she'd be just fine in menopause. After all, her mother had six children, and even she was fine! (Now she thinks her mother was probably suffering but soldiering on.)

So Liz was surprised by how hard the transition hit her: "In perimenopause, I gained so much weight, about sixty pounds. I've also always been such a sexual person, and all of a sudden everything became unbalanced. Sometimes I was really feeling it and wanting it, even more than I did in my twenties. And then other times, nothing. I was not interested at all. In fact, I began to obsess about gardening, and unlike my mom, I hated gardening! I also obsessed about food. When I had sex, I'd look over the man's shoulder and think, *I want a pizza*. And I started to imagine it while I was having sex: sizzling pepperoni pizza. Eventually I didn't want sex at all. That part of me was dead."

Liz heard about HRT and wondered if it might be good for her, so she went to a doctor. But because her mother had died of breast cancer at sixty-seven and the doctor wasn't trained in menopause, the doctor said, "Absolutely not." This is even though Liz didn't have the BRCA gene.

One doctor even told her, "When are women going to just accept the rhythm of life? You have your teenage years, you have your twenties and your thirties, and you have children, and now you're going into another part of life."

How infuriating is that? This vibrant, sexual woman was suffering, and the doctor was patting her on the hand and telling her to just suck it up!

Finally, she researched hormones on her own and realized that they would most likely be safe for her. She found a new doctor, who put her on low-dose HRT, and she couldn't believe how much better she felt.

"My clit was pounding again!" Liz said. "When a man calls, I'm wet just having a discussion. I'm seventy years old, and what I want younger women to know is that life doesn't have to end with menopause. I am so full of life. More than you could ever imagine. My theme is to say yes to everything. I'm confident in how I look. I learned to focus on being generous, giving, loving. When you look around and stop obsessing inwardly, you feel so full of life. I have a phone that blows up with sexts from a man I want. I'm up for any adventure at the drop of a hat. I'm living my best life. I've earned it."

By this age, we've had our share of experiences, both good and bad, and we've learned from both. We're not being governed by our desire to reproduce or our fear of becoming pregnant. We're willing to say, "Yeah, no, don't put your hand there. Put your hand *here.*"

I do think women sometimes become more sexual as they get older because they know themselves and they lose the awkwardness of youth. You might need to be more organized—once again, you may need a lubricant within reach—but the more comfortable we are with ourselves and the more we know what we want, the more we can tell our partners about it and the more pleasurable sex becomes for everyone. There's something so liberating about working through hard truths and freeing yourself from shame.

Things They Really Should Tell Us About Sex in Menopause

- Sex drive often goes down at this age, but the female corollary to erectile dysfunction, hypoactive sexual desire disorder (HSDD), is fully treatable.

- The Female Sexual Function Index measures six areas: desire, arousal, lubrication, orgasm, satisfaction, and pain. A woman might have issues in anywhere from none to all six of these areas.

- There is a natural, normal gap between a male and a female partner when it comes to reaching orgasm. For women, the average time from the start of a sexual encounter to orgasm is four to ten minutes on our own, ten to twenty minutes with a partner. It's also very common to need something instead of or in addition to penetrative intercourse for women to orgasm.

- Urine leakage, frequent UTIs, and vaginal dryness can all contribute to reduced sexual responses, and local estrogen cream can help with all these things.

- "Use it or lose it" is bunk. The myth came from a study that showed correlation between more sex and the absence of pain with sex, not causality. It's insanity to tell women that they should have sex to prevent a hormonal change that might be causing sex to be more painful.

- Vaginal estrogen can help with many symptoms of hyposexual desire disorder. Lifestyle changes can make a difference, too, as can testosterone (in the correct dosage!). Communication is often a major factor in sexual pleasure for women.

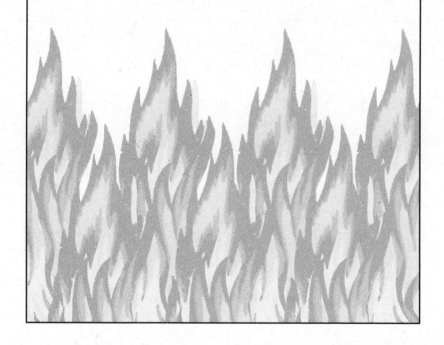

CHAPTER FOUR

SHAME

S hame—such a big subject. Where do we begin with this one? Constant comparison started for me at puberty. As a girl of twelve, I, like my brother, went to boarding school. Living full-time with about thirty other girls, I became extremely conscious of how slowly I was developing. There was spoken and unspoken competition among the girls: *Who has the biggest boobs? Who's stuffing tissues in their bra? Who has their period? Who's made out with someone? Who has pubic hair?* We were like detectives trying to solve a murder mystery. We spent hours talking about all of these things, vibrating with anticipation. I was always dead last to every milestone, and I lived in fear that everyone would find out.

I was fourteen and not yet menstruating. The only other girl besides me for whom this was true was a friend of mine. Until one day she came running up to me saying, "I got it! It's come!" My heart sank. Was I to be left completely alone in the trenches?

"No, you don't have your period!" I said to my friend. "I bet you don't. Don't leave me all alone in this!"

"I do, though!" she said. "Come, look!"

She pulled me into the bathroom and showed me her soaked sanitary towel, as we used to call them then.

"Oh my God; it's true," I said, as if I'd been given terrible news.

The sight of that pad sent me into a panic: this meant I was going to be undesirable and had failed at becoming a woman! The party of adulthood was in full swing, and I alone hadn't received an invitation. I thought, *I've got to somehow be a part of this. I have to.*

So I did what I thought would make me a part of the club: I bought myself a box of tampons. Then I locked myself in the bathroom and spent a good forty-five minutes stuffing one into my not-yet-bleeding vagina. I certainly did not have my period, but when I changed clothes or got out of the shower, I wanted any girl who looked at me to see the string and know that I was One of Them.

In my experience, there is little about being a girl or woman that shame does not touch. Some of the things we might feel shame about: not having gotten a period yet or having too heavy a period. Having a C-section, getting an epidural, not breastfeeding, not having babies at all, having too many babies. Not working enough or working too much. Too girly, too scary. Too wet, too dry. Too petite, too womanly. Too ambitious, too lazy. Too slutty, too frigid. Caring too much about how you look, not caring enough. . . . Gah!

We kept so many secrets from one another when we were young, and why? I learned how to masturbate from *Cosmopolitan* and spent a whole summer reading smutty scenes in Sidney Sheldon books though I felt far too awkward to speak about it with a friend. How much information and solace we could have provided to one another if we hadn't been so anxious about random time lines, so obsessed with what being early or late meant for our romantic prospects, so *scared*.

I look back now and see the irony of my time at boarding school. We spend the first part of our lives trying to be more mature and older. Then at some point along the way the question becomes *How do I look younger? How do I stay youthful?*

This feeling of always being the wrong age followed me to Hollywood. Why have I always felt too young or too old but never exactly the right age? For so long, I was the youngest person on set. I've since become one of the oldest. Why have I never, not once in decades of filming, felt smack in the middle? For a long time, I was afraid to talk about menopause, and I secretly took hormones, not mentioning it even to people I was close with. Slowly I started to try to talk about it, making jokes with my friends about estrogen dips and things like that. I kept trying to come up with a cute way of saying I was in menopause without actually saying it. But as I tested the waters, the admission was often met with nervous laughter or "Oh, don't be silly. This is far too early for menopause." Confirmation that my body had failed. The shame deepened.

It wasn't good for me to live that way. I was deeply affected by not having an outlet for my fears and feelings. I was lonely. Just as

I'd felt I couldn't speak openly about infertility, now, a few years later, I felt that I had to keep secret my struggles with menopause. It became a kind of monster in the closet.

I grappled with questions about my self-worth: *Can I still play leading ladies?* Menopause didn't feel like just the end of menstruation. It felt like the end of *everything*: fertility, sexuality, vibrancy— and my ability to be honest with other people about what was going on with me.

Carrying that kind of burden is not sustainable, but for so long I didn't know how to explain how sensitive I was and how I still didn't understand what was going on.

When I called menopause expert Dr. Jen Gunter to ask for her thoughts on shame, she said it's connected to everything about being a woman: "Pretty much everything I deal with in my job is filled with shame, which is really sad. I see people with vaginal health problems, and they think that their vaginas stink, and I see people with vulva problems, and they think their vulvas are ugly. And then I see people feeling completely invisible or shameful because they're going through menopause.

"And I would say that those fears seem perfectly normal to me in the society that we're in. You're only of value to the patriarchy if you're a breeder. And then when you finish breeding, you need to shut up and go away. And by the way, you need to be a breeder with a tight vagina because men don't understand how vaginas work. If your mother grew up in that system, and her mother grew up in that system, and *her* mother grew up in that system back and back and back and back, then we've been steeping in it for centuries. You and I are not that far removed from it being pretty bad."

I agree with her. In my industry, you see so many male stars in their forties and fifties with twenty-four-year-old girlfriends. "We see all the women on television look a certain way," Dr. Gunter said. "We're fed these messages about virginity, and this idea that once you're done being of use to men, you're just chucked in the pile. I mean, it's no different than in *The Handmaid's Tale*. Your value is as a wife, as a mother, not as a person. I've been in department meetings where I was told I needed to seek psychiatric care for getting upset over something. I wasn't crying, wasn't screaming. I was just saying, 'This is unacceptable.'"

Generally older women in movies and on TV were always acting out, being a bit crazy. Not that this isn't often to great comic effect. I always enjoyed the British TV comedy show *Absolutely Fabulous*. God, the two over-the-top middle-aged women who starred in it were hilarious, and though I would have hated to be the put-upon daughter in the story, I just loved the characters of Edina and Patsy. (I related to the mousy daughter, Saffy, because I was shy and my mother was bold—she showed up to one assembly in tight leather pants and platform boots, and I know she wouldn't mind my telling you that she could be a bit mouthy.)

We look outward to determine what's "normal." And then there's almost no limit to what we will do to ourselves to try to feel normal, to combat the loneliness and the shame of our bodies not matching the bodies of the women we see around us. That insecurity and isolation starts young, and for me, like a shame bookend, it hit again when I became menopausal. Historically, menopause was considered so shameful that people didn't even call it by name but instead used euphemisms: "the change," "second spring," "private summer," "ovarian retirement."

Too often, doctors lack proper training and so decide their struggling patients are just tired, depressed, or delusional. This is one major contributing factor in so many women's painful journey of shame in menopause—because they felt like hypochondriacs or couldn't get the support they needed, they turned inward and retreated.

For many months I suffered from a shoulder that wouldn't rotate all the way and caused me pain. I assumed it would go away on its own one day, but after a full year of consistent pain, physical therapy, and talking to friends who had the same thing, I went to a doctor. I explained that it was keeping me up at night and had been going on for a long time.

An MRI was ordered. When it came back the doctor said, "How did you injure yourself?"

"I didn't injure myself," I said. "It came on a year ago and hasn't gotten better. I've heard from friends who've had this that it could be related to menopause. They say there's something called 'frozen shoulder,' and—"

"Okay, it's adhesive capsulitis, but let's get you a cortisone shot and see if it helps," the doctor said with a patronizing smile. He seemed to think it was cute that I thought I knew better than he did. His tone: *Who was I to question a medical expert?*

Next doctor, younger than the first one, same thing. He smiled and looked uncomfortable when I said the word "menopause," so I was immediately also uncomfortable. While I didn't expect him or the first guy to know much about this condition, since menopause wasn't their specialty, I didn't expect to be questioned as if I was a child: "Are you sure you didn't injure yourself and just forget?"

But with the second doctor, who appeared to be closer in age to my children than to me, I pushed. I insisted he look up "menopause" and "frozen shoulder." I said, "Why wouldn't there be a possible connection? There are estrogen receptors all over the body. The demographic that gets frozen shoulder most commonly is women aged forty to sixty. A dozen of my friends have it, too."

He told me he hadn't heard of such a connection and that it sounded anecdotal. He seemed to think of me as what I'm told doctors sometimes call us when we complain: a "ww," for "whiny woman." (For the record, I think the shot did help, though four months later, I started to feel a dull pain when I was in bed.)

The patriarchy has limited doctors' education about how menopause affects the entire body. The gender health gap is vast. If we're going to keep from sinking into shame, a whole lot more shifting is needed. Women have to help change the narrative. Don't suffer. Don't expect pain. Ask for help. So what if, because of their ignorance, the doctors think you're ridiculous? *You're* paying *them*. It's their job to take you seriously even if they suspect you're wrong.

Another arena for shaming: sex, especially a desire to enjoy it. Some women pushed into menopause by cancer treatment complain of painful sex and are essentially told, "You should feel grateful you're alive."

Can you imagine? As though a woman should be ashamed of wanting to enjoy that life fully!

"The vast majority of patients I treat are women who have breast cancer and are also bothered by changes to their sexual function after their cancer treatment," said Dr. Stacy Lindau. "Now, if a woman with breast cancer is not already in menopause when she goes through cancer treatment, regardless of her age, the chemo will very likely trigger menopause. And it's oftentimes a much more abrupt onset and extreme set of symptoms. It's not uncommon for women to present with extreme dryness, irritation in the genital area, both externally in the vulva and internally in the vagina, loss of sensation in their clitoris, even—in women taking anti-hormone therapy—flattening of the clitoris or the feeling of *Where did my clitoris go?*

"Imagine that we treated men in midlife with a medicine that was going to cause their penis to shrink up or be unrecognizable. Doctors would *mention this*, and by the way, men would never take this drug. But with women, we've done very little to track the impact of these drugs on the size, the volume, the sensitivity of the clitoris, to even counsel women in an evidence-based way. But more than fifteen years I've been seeing women with breast cancer on aromatase inhibitors. And so I have good empirical evidence from my clinical practice about what happens."

Let's pause for a moment to point out that early menopause is triggered in so many women being treated for cancer and that they then have to cope with sexual health problems. And, again, they may have to do this while being told they should just be happy they survived!

Similarly, I think so many women have birth trauma but are told just to be grateful they wound up with a healthy baby. After my Cesarean, I wept because I hadn't managed to birth my baby "the natural way" and I was left with a gaping wound in my body. I was so determined to have a natural birth the second time that I fired my OB at thirty-six weeks when she said she was just placating me by talking about a VBAC (a vaginal birth following a C-section). With my new doctor I wound up with yet another traumatic birth, which led me to a baby in the NICU for three days, with me thinking it was all my fault.

Fortunately, I've begun in all areas of my life to care so much less about what people think. Perhaps because I finally realized that feeling ashamed is *exhausting,* and I don't have the energy to spare. Speaking with friends; speaking with Billy, who's been so understanding; and then speaking publicly about my experience has alleviated my shame and given me the ability to shrug when faced with the reality of my menopausal body.

This became clear to me one day at the drugstore. I was picking up my HRT, as well as a prescription for a UTI and an over-the-counter cream for a yeast infection. During checkout, the pharmacist started announcing it all on the speakerphone, "Price check: Aisle Four, the Vaginal Care section . . ."

Oh my God, I thought, feeling the way I had when I bought tampons as a teenager. The pharmacists loudly discussed my Vagisil purchase as a queue formed behind me.

When I turned to leave, I saw a dad from my kid's school. I noticed him a second before he noticed me, so I looked away, hoping he'd take the hint and leave me alone with what the whole store now knew to be my distressed vagina.

He did not.

"Naomi, great to see you! How are you doing?" he said.

Uh, after all that, I think you know how I'm doing, Ted.

But what the hell? If he didn't know about middle-aged women's bodies, maybe he should.

"Doing fine, Ted, thanks," I said. "And I'll be better now that I've picked up these meds. Good to see you, too."

Things They Really Should Tell Us About Shame

- We compare ourselves to other women to the detriment of all. One upside of menopause is that these comparisons often end. And if we're able to speak openly about the complexity of our experience, we can end them even sooner.

- We all have problems with our bodies from time to time; that doesn't mean we're broken or have anything to be embarrassed about when we need help.

- Middle-aged women often go through a period of feeling invisible, which makes sense in a society where women's value is so closely tied to a narrow idea of beauty, sexuality, and reproduction.

- We can trust ourselves on so many things, and we can learn to advocate for our own health.

- Keeping secrets is exhausting. "Coming out" as being menopausal can help evaporate any shame you feel, and it will help others shed shame as well.

CHAPTER FIVE

ANXIETY, RAGE, PANIC, DEPRESSION, GRIEF

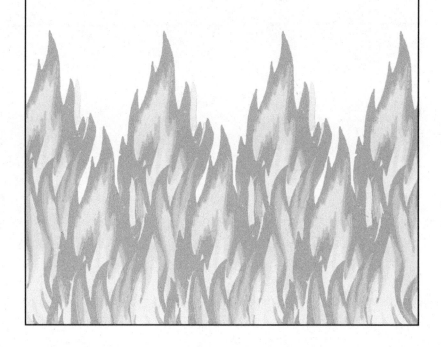

They say menopause is like puberty in reverse, and for many of us there's a sort of mirror experience of those early days. It's no wonder, because hormone fluctuation is directly linked to mood, and in both times of life it's common to have harrowing emotional highs and lows.

One woman now on the other side of menopause and thriving told me that she'd spent a few years being miserable: "I had really dramatic hot flashes that felt sort of like panic attacks or rage attacks. They felt like *panicky rage*. I wanted out of my skin, and I wanted to *kick things*. Often, I felt that I wanted to take all my clothes off and kick the oven. We were in a tiny apartment, and I kept hiding from my kids in my closet because I was so angry, and I didn't want to show them that part of me."

Another recalled her mother's intense experience of menopause: "One night she threw a raw chicken at me. An *entire chicken*."

I was moved to learn that the anxiety-rage-panic cycle even came to Dr. Suzanne Gilberg-Lenz. She told me it happened to her in her midforties: "I was an insane person," she said. "I'd never had PMS. And then, all of a sudden, I was enraged, really dark. It was not good. My medical assistant confessed that everybody in the office knew my cycle, just by how I was acting. And *I* didn't know."

Like me, Dr. Gilberg-Lenz hadn't been prepared by her elders: "My mom was the best, but my mom's from the fifties. She didn't tell me anything. I had no idea. And when I started sharing with patients what I'd learned and how it might be connected to mood symptoms they were experiencing I sometimes heard, 'This can't be happening to me!' As if I told them they had cancer. 'It can't be *menopause*!' Like that was going to kill them somehow."

During a snack break at a menopause conference Stripes Beauty organized with The Swell, Dr. Ellen Vora, who practices holistic psychiatry and is the author of *The Anatomy of Anxiety*, offered some perspective. "These perimenopausal and postmenopausal years are a perfect storm for mental health," she said. "What I see is astronomical rates of anxiety—and for good reason. The hormonal shift directly impacts mental health, but it also compromises our sleep, which in turn contributes to depression and anxiety. Then you add to that all of the role transitions we go through at this age—we may be sandwiched between raising young children and grappling with aging parents, then we have teenagers in the house, and then an empty nest to contend with. Meanwhile, we're perceived differently by our culture, which values youth above all else. So we come by our rising rates of depression and anxiety honestly.

"It looks different in everybody. One person might have generalized anxiety disorder, like a chronic low-grade state of worry and tension. Another might have panic attacks out of the blue or develop agoraphobic symptoms. In someone else, it could be an exacerbation of social anxiety symptoms. A lot of people have a combination of different symptoms. That's not to mention the uptick of depression as well."

I asked her if she saw what I'd seen: we go to our doctors with all these symptoms, and we're handed a script for Prozac or Lexapro or Celexa and sent on our way. "Oh, yes. Part of the problem is that practitioners have so little time—usually only eight to fifteen minutes with a patient. They're overwhelmed and running behind, and they're hardly trained to hold space for messy emotions.

"So, if you go in and mention that you're feeling more anxious or depressed—or, God forbid, you start to cry—your doctor is thinking, *how do I solve this problem in the seven minutes that remain?* What choice do they have but to write a prescription?

"Another reason doctors are quick to offer an antidepressant for menopausal symptoms," Dr. Vora says, "is that Western medicine has a fundamentally flawed understanding of mental health. We're operating according to the 'monoamine hypothesis of depression and anxiety.' That's the idea that our mental health issues are the result of a genetic chemical imbalance. If we're depressed or anxious, it's because we have low serotonin. This is not only our least hopeful understanding of mental health—it's also wrong."

Dr. Vora is one doctor who's pushing for broader definitions: "Large meta-analyses have revealed that, for mild to moderate depression, an antidepressant doesn't differ much from placebo. When it works, it's great. But for the unlucky majority who don't experience sufficient relief from symptoms, it can leave people feeling hopeless and despairing."

Dr. Vora continues:

In menopause, when shifts in estrogen and progesterone are the true root cause of depression and anxiety, psychiatric medications, aimed at serotonin, are barking up the wrong tree. We are more likely to find enduring relief from symptoms by addressing the underlying root causes, whether that means hormone replacement or lifestyle modifications to support sleep, nutrition, inflammation, movement, gut health, or stress. Often it's important to address our psycho-spiritual needs as well, such as carving out space to grieve, addressing unresolved trauma, and reconnecting to community.

When we shift our narrative away from mental health as a genetic chemical destiny and toward a "growth mindset" view of mental health—that our mental health can improve, that we're never stuck, and that there are safe and accessible ways we can support ourselves—we can feel empowered and hopeful, and we can finally experience lasting relief from symptoms.

Dr. Vora is tapping into a bigger conversation going on right now about antidepressants as possibly having been oversold as cure-alls. It's controversial, but what I think we can all agree on is that we should be offered a full range of options, medical and otherwise.

Dr. Vora said that, while some people do suffer from debilitating depression that only medication touches, in some cases, supporting our own mental health is within our grasp.

Step one is figuring out exactly what's wrong. Dr. Vora explained that "we have false and true anxiety. False anxiety is anxiety based in the body, and it's *avoidable*—it's the anxiety that comes from skipping breakfast, or from drinking too much coffee, from sleep deprivation, and from a hangover. Once you fix the root cause—keeping blood sugar stable, moderating caffeine intake, prioritizing sleep, and taking more nights off from drinking—false anxiety goes away." There are many small, actionable strategies we can try. Many of Dr. Vora's patients take a spoonful of coconut oil or almond butter a few times a day to stabilize blood sugar, supplement with magnesium glycinate, and support sleep by taking a morning walk in the sun and then wearing glasses that filter out blue light after sunset.

True anxiety, on the other hand, is not a "problem." Dr. Vora said, "It's actually what's *right* with us when we're able to viscerally connect to what's wrong in the world around us. It's not something to pathologize—it's something to listen to. I think of true anxiety as an electric fence, nudging us back into alignment when we need a course correction. In order to hear the clarion call of our true anxiety, we first need to address our false anxiety (otherwise we will confuse a blood sugar crash for our deep inner truth), and then we need to slow down, be still, and listen. Helpful practices can be meditation, breathwork, journaling, spending time in nature, and my personal favorite: having a good cry." She adds, "We all carry so much unprocessed, unmetabolized grief."

I was glad she brought up grief. Grief doesn't get talked about nearly enough, as far as I'm concerned. So many of us at this age have had reason to mourn, whether it's the loss of a job or a relationship or a pregnancy or our children leaving home or our parents dying or our friends getting sick or a thousand other things. Many women I know have confessed to me that they feel they have lost themselves, too. "Have I become the terminally unhip mom in teen comedies?" a friend asked me recently. Crying is often an appropriate response to what we're going through.

The novelist Sigrid Nunez, who won the National Book Award for *The Friend* (I appear in the film adaptation), writes beautifully about grief and how to embrace it. She says that we may have deep sorrow over who we might have been and what life we might have had. But it's not a tragedy, feeling grief. It just means we're human.

Speaking at the Chicago Humanities Festival, Nunez said something profound: that reckoning with what we have and don't have in midlife leads to "a certain kind of mournfulness about life, even in people who are optimistic and generally happy. Sometimes that unexplained sadness feels like grief. Part of it is for your father who died ten years ago and that grief never really left you, but I also think that it's mourning for other things you've lost. . . . Life creates a certain amount of bereavement with every day that you live. You store it up. It becomes part of you. You can't let that take over, because that's when you despair, which is what you don't want to do. You want to find the strength to live with grief without denying it."

And one way you handle it and live with it without denying it? Cry! Cry as much as you can! Dr. Vora calls crying "free therapy."

Oh, but it took me so long to become okay with crying unless I was being paid to on camera! Remember, I grew up in England and Australia, where visible emotion of any kind was frowned upon and we had to keep "a stiff upper lip"—absurd, I know!

And don't even get my fellow Brits started on therapy! That was considered indulgent or navel gazing. There was a stigma from my grandparents' generation that therapy was only for "crazy people." And we weren't allowed to sit around reading books, for that matter. *That was lazy! There were animals to feed, pens to clean! No one had time to be depressed!*

So I was definitely a reluctant therapy patient. I'd tell myself: *What have you got to complain about? Suck it up!* My mum at her midlife point rejected cultural norms and started getting into different kinds of New Age-y forms of self-examination. You can imagine my reaction as a teenager was that therapy felt a bit wacky. Let's say I'm pretty sure I was rolling my eyes—like I catch my kids doing when I talk about menopause or sexual health, or when I breathe too loudly.

But in the years since I came to America, I've slowly changed. From my early forties onward, I've become quite serious about therapy and about other ways to feel better, including meditation, yoga, and exercise. I've been persuaded of the value of not only regular journaling but "future journaling"—writing about how you want the future to look. I've learned how to take myself out of situations that make me anxious. I used to be obsessive about filling out my dance card, but now I feel okay about missing things. I'm still very social, but I've become much less so. I hate going out midweek if I can avoid it. I need to be up early with the kids, and anything that will interfere with seven hours of sleep is a nonstarter. I say no to things I don't want to do—and even no to things I do want to do sometimes. I stay away from people who drain me.

I keep up boundaries, and I take breaks. When the kids are being rude or behaving in a way that bumps me to the point of easy escalation, I take myself for a walk with the dog—"I'm taking Izzy for a walk to go and get milk!"—in the hope that some fresh air and a time-out will let me cool off and reset. I let myself recover from busy weeks. I follow the rhythms of my interest and let there be ups and downs.

As I've sought balance in my social life, I've found that hormone therapy has helped keep me on an even emotional keel. Many women find HRT helpful for mood swings, and it also helps with sleep, which is a major cause of emotional volatility. I'd never presume to tell other women what to do with their bodies, but I do want them to know that there's no reason to dismiss hormone therapy out of hand if it's safe for you, and there's also no reason to suffer.

Of course, this better quality of life can be available in other ways, too. One is just getting through to the other side of the menopausal transition. So many women report feeling way better once they're no longer menstruating—a reclaiming, a return to themselves.

The woman I mentioned earlier who had the "panicky rage"— one doctor put her on antidepressants. "That did help even me out, but they made me feel a little bit sick and I gained weight."

She tried many different treatments, from supplements to expensive creams, and nothing was working for her. She had the antidrug philosophy shared by another woman I know: "I felt like everyone else should be taking drugs to make *them* less annoying to *me*." So she developed a new game plan.

She said: "I'm going to go off absolutely everything. I'm going to really pay attention to my sleep, my nutrition, and my overall health." It took a few months, but she began to see a change, and then a few more months to feel fully out of the woods. Within a year she'd found her way out of hell, and she stopped hiding in her closet.

For some women, lifestyle changes are enough to get back on track. For others, hormone therapy is the path back to feeling good. In the next two chapters I'm going to talk about when it might be worth considering hormones and, if you decide HRT is something you want to do, how it all works.

Things They Really Should Tell Us About Mood Swings

- Not all anxiety is bad. There's a difference between false anxiety and true anxiety.

- One of the first steps to dealing with mood swings should be stabilizing blood sugar and getting enough sleep.

- Depression is not just about inherited brain chemistry. There might be other factors like work stress, loneliness, or a lack of community.

- Antidepressants work for some people—and I have a lot of friends who feel they have been profoundly helped by them—but they are not game changers for everyone.

- Unprocessed grief is real. There's a lot of mourning to do at this age. Crying is free therapy.

CHAPTER SIX

IS HORMONE THERAPY SAFE?

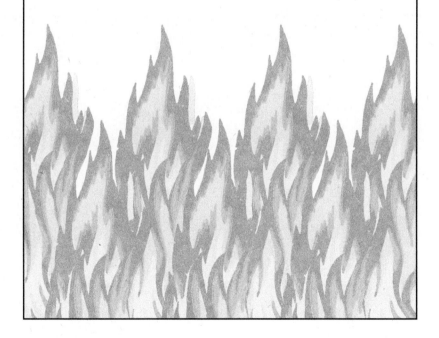

N ow, finally, we come to the practical question of what we can actually do to address the most severe menopause symptoms. The questions around hormone replacement therapy (HRT) are some of the most consistently fraught ones, not just for us menopausal women but even among doctors—as I found when I tried to reconcile all my favorite experts' opinions in this chapter! The number of opinions can really make your head spin—and not like watching a calm tennis match, but more like Linda Blair's head swiveling in *The Exorcist*. The whole time I was writing this chapter, I kept hearing conflicting information.

What I've chosen to do is to present the positions of a number of doctors whom I trust and to name the places where they disagree. When it comes to our health, we have to weigh so many different factors. I hope sharing my story and my research will help you make your own decisions (in consultation with your doctor, of course!).

By the time I was in my early forties, I was experiencing regular night sweats and hot flashes, but I told no one. I felt lucky that at least I wasn't having them every day. Still, I was desperate for symptom relief. And yet, I found myself confused about hormones in general and hormone therapy specifically—would HRT kill me or save my life? Either option felt so extreme. I was not afraid of hormones per se, as I'd been on birth control for a large portion of my life and understood that women sometimes used it as a way to control early symptoms of menopause. Still, I kept wondering: *Where is the middle ground?* So far in this book I've been talking about using hormones for relief of various symptoms; now, let's get down to the basics, because there is a lot of misinformation out there.

Hormones are essentially chemicals that act as messengers throughout the body to tell cells and organs to behave in certain ways. When I first learned about how many aspects of the female body are linked to hormones—mood, hair growth, mental health, sleep, digestion, lust, fertility, basically everything—the overall experience of menopause started to make more sense.

To complicate things even more, menopause is not one size fits all. Some women have terrible perimenopausal symptoms for many years, whereas some never have any. Some women approaching menopause have years of superheavy periods that soak through their clothes, and others have periods that become lighter than when they first began menstruating. Some women have ten hot flashes a day, and others never have a single one.

Here's a typical story from one friend of mine: "After six months of menopause symptoms and no periods, I got what can only be described as the fucking heaviest period of my life. It was insane. I was so depleted of iron that I started eating liver. I got another period three weeks later, and another one four weeks later, and then the following month. And I'm like, *Okay, what's happening now? Is my period back?* Now, my menopause symptoms have gone away. These are the things no one tells you."

When a woman starts experiencing hot flashes, she might go for tests to determine her average hormone levels thinking she'll learn how much longer symptoms are likely to last. That's when she learns that there's no one test to determine if she's in menopause. I'm told there are some emerging over-the-counter products that check hormone levels but that it's still unclear how to best make use of them. Endocrinologist Dr. Rocio Salas-Whalen says, "The drop of estrogen during this transition is not a linear, steep drop. It's more like a roller coaster, with estrogen levels up and down in no specific order or time. Due to this, it's difficult to diagnose perimenopause based on labs." And so we can spend years in this netherworld, not sure where we are in the menopause journey and therefore not sure what to do about symptom relief and contraception.

One of the more arduous detours I went on in the course of getting proper treatment happened in 2013. I'd been filming in

Mozambique. A few months later, back in the United States, I needed to show vaccination paperwork because I wanted to volunteer for a school excursion. I needed a booster for TB. When I got that vaccination, my arm blew up. It got more and more agitated and swollen. I ended up going to the ER. The doctor thought I might have had some sort of infection. Because I'd ticked "night sweats" and "migraines" on my intake form, my doctor thought tuberculosis was a possibility. Then when I tested borderline positive for TB (which I later learned can happen after a booster), everyone freaked out. I was given chest X-rays and a massive blood workup. The tests went on for weeks until it was confirmed that I did not, in fact, have TB. But, again, the perimenopause-related symptoms just sat there on my chart, completely missed!

Now that I'm much more informed, here is my rough explanation of what generally happens in our bodies when we enter perimenopause: Our levels of estrogen and progesterone (the hormones produced by the ovaries after ovulation to sustain a pregnancy) start fluctuating. Levels of testosterone (which has been proven to be beneficial to orgasm, arousal, and pleasure) that have been declining for decades before menopause keep declining. Meanwhile, we see a rise in the levels of follicle-stimulating hormone (FSH), the hormone that signals when to ovulate.

In menopause, when your estrogen drops, your FSH goes up. If your FSH level is consistently over 30 international units per liter, that's one sign of menopause. (A typical range for a woman who's still fertile is around 5 to 21.) However, menopause is confirmed by an elevated FSH only once you've also had one full year without-periods.

It can all be so confusing—even for me, and I've had more hormone tests than I care to admit. Although I was still bleeding in my late thirties while I was trying to conceive, my FSH levels kept merrily bouncing around in the twenties, thirties, and forties—the menopausal range. But until I had a full year without a period, my being in menopause wasn't "official."

If I'd been middle-aged in the 1990s or in the three decades before, I likely would have been offered relief from the symptoms of menopause: HRT, which would have offered my body estrogen and progesterone (or other progestogens); or, if I had had a hysterectomy, I would have been offered estrogen replacement therapy (ERT) alone.

These hormones can be given as pills, gels, sprays, a vaginal ring, or patches. Which version you get might be determined by certain health concerns, cost, availability, or personal preference. The version you take will also be guided by where in menopause you are. Some tips on language: "Systemic" means you take hormones that travel through your entire body and treat the symptoms of menopause. "Local" means you apply the hormones in one place, like putting estrogen cream in your vagina or topical estrogen on your face. These are low doses, and there is no significant increase in your blood levels of estrogen.

If you're perimenopausal and don't need birth control or have cycle-control issues, you may be given "cyclical HRT" (meaning you take estrogen every day but progesterone only part of the month). With cyclical HRT you may continue to have periods. Another option you might be offered in perimenopause is a hormone-based IUD like Mirena with estrogen therapy. It provides progesterone and protects the uterus from cancer, often decreases or stops bleeding, and provides birth control. (I've found that a lot of women are reluctant to stop their periods entirely if they're still having them. Which I understand! Letting go entirely can feel like a massive shift, identity-wise. It makes sense to want to hold on to what can feel like a last vestige of youth.)

If it's been a year or more since you've had a period, you'll more likely be given "continuous HRT," which means you'll take both estrogen and progesterone every day. Women who've had a hysterectomy are able to take estrogen alone. Other women are prescribed a combination of estrogen and progesterone, which protects the uterine lining, to lessen the risk of endometrial cancer.

While HRT doesn't reverse menopause, it can help a woman get through this time without feeling the worst effects of declining estrogen. Usually hot flashes go away in less than two weeks, and it may take six to eight weeks for the other benefits to kick in. Within three months or so you get the full effect, potentially including (in some women) improvements to heart health, sexual function, memory, and vaginal health.

Confirming these benefits, a major study published in spring of 2024 by the *Journal of the American Medical Association* said generally hormone therapy is safe as a treatment for relief of menopause symptoms below the age of sixty. To understand the study better, I called Dr. JoAnn E. Manson, the Michael and Lee Bell Professor of Women's Health at Harvard Medical School, former head of the Menopause Society, and first author of the study.

"There's tremendous variability in women's symptoms and quality of life issues," she told me. "Many women can be relatively free of symptoms through menopause and treatment would not be indicated. They are having minimal symptoms, they're not having disrupted sleep, they're not having really bothersome hot flashes, night sweats. Then there are women who have very distressing symptoms, having ten or fifteen hot flashes every day and being awakened frequently with night sweats, and their sleep is very disrupted. And that can lead to poorer quality of life and other problems. Of course, if sleep is being constantly disrupted, there will be difficulties with concentration, there will be brain fog, there can be mood changes and depression."

Side effects of HRT can include aching breasts or headaches, though they usually get milder or go away within a few months. "But it's also not good for health to have disrupted sleep," Dr. Manson said. "It's not good for health to have impaired quality of life and the stress that comes with that. So as an overall trade-off, for a woman in early menopause with bothersome or distressing menopausal symptoms, HRT would make sense unless she's at a very high baseline risk of breast cancer, cardiovascular disease, or has other major risk factors." Nonetheless, many women who don't have a high risk of developing cancer are scared to try HRT because there's been a lot of misinformation about the cancer risk. I, too, was concerned about potential risks when I began my research. But ultimately after my doctor walked me through the risks and benefits I was convinced that it was right for me.

Here's why: HRT was regularly offered starting in the 1960s, and it became even more popular in the 1990s. Then, in 2002, something dramatic happened: a branch of the Women's Health Initiative's long-term hormone replacement therapy study was abruptly stopped. This was first announced not via a journal article but rather by a widely covered surprise press conference (about a week before the publication) with a message that boiled down to a misleading headline: "HRT = Breast Cancer and Other Major Health Risks!"

Medical oncologist Dr. Avrum Bluming and social psychologist Dr. Carol Tavris have been researching hormones for decades. They are coauthors of the book *Estrogen Matters: Why Taking Hormones in Menopause Can Improve Women's Well-Being and Lengthen Their Lives—Without Raising the Risk of Breast Cancer*. Dr. Tavris told me, "On the day of the WHI press conference, I don't think I'd even had a cup of coffee yet before the phone rang. It was Avrum. He was on the ceiling: *Have you seen this press conference?*"

So many doctors were caught off guard by the flood of worried calls to their offices. That shocking moment caused a pullback in menopause research and treatment with effects we're still feeling today.

Women, including my mother, immediately started flushing their hormone pills down the toilet. In the years that followed, I'd notice her sneaking pills here and there. And I remember saying, "What is that?" And she would say, "It's HRT. It's not really safe anymore, but it makes me feel good." She'd allow herself a treat for a few special days to get that little oomph back in her system.

Dr. Bluming told me:

At the time we got interested in this area, the mid-1980s moving into the 1990s, estrogen was used widely. The numbers vary depending upon what you read, but approximately 44 percent of eligible menopausal women were taking hormones. And then on July 8, 2002, the press conference of the Women's Health Initiative investigators was held, and around the Western world, that number fell to less than 5 percent. And it has stayed in that area now for more than twenty years.

Yes, as with any medication, there are risks with HRT, including gallstones and blood clots. According to Dr. Rocio Salas-Whalen: "The reason for the blood clot risk with oral estradiol is that it's broken down in the liver and this can start the clotting cascade. Transdermal estradiol, on the other hand, is metabolized in the kidney, lessening the risk of blood clots." She also notes, "Obesity and age are independent risk factors for the development of gallstones, which might increase the risk in women in this age group.

The WHI reported that HRT increases the risk of stroke. However, the increase in stroke only occurred in women starting hormones for the first time after the age of sixty-five, and only for the first year of use. After the first year, the risk returns to baseline. The risk of blood clots, too, is higher for the first year and then goes back to normal.

To give a sense of how high the health risk is from taking HRT: the greatest danger is a gallbladder event. In one study, 8 out of every 1,000 women per year taking hormones had gallbladder problems compared with about 5 in every 1,000 women per year for those taking a placebo. So HRT multiplies your risk by about 1.6, but those chances are still quite remote. And the odds for developing the other issues are even lower.

"Hormones don't increase the risk of heart disease and heart death," Dr. Bluming told me. "They *decrease* the risk of heart disease and heart death. They don't increase the risk of cognitive decline; they *decrease* the risk of cognitive decline. They also help prevent hip fractures, from which approximately as many older women die in the first year as die of breast cancer. We now know that estrogen-only treatment decreases the risk of developing breast cancer by 23 percent and decreases the risk of death from breast cancer by 40 percent."

What else didn't make it into the press? Among the women taking estrogen alone because they'd had hysterectomies, there was *no* increased risk of breast cancer. (About one in three women have this surgery before age sixty, often to stop heavy periods caused by fibroids or because of uterine prolapse, endometriosis, or cancer.)

The one thing the WHI is still claiming is that the combination of estrogen and progestin given to women who still have a uterus does increase the risk of breast cancer development. "But even that small increase," Dr. Bluming points out, "misrepresents and inflates the WHI's own data."

Those who maintain that the data supports a slight uptick in breast cancer risk say it's not nothing, but most now grant that it's far from as strong a correlation as many of us had been led to believe. What I find interesting is that there are so many other HRT options that have never been associated with those sorts of risks. For instance, women who don't want to be on systemic estrogen for whatever reason can use vaginal estrogen, which is just applied locally—or they can try vaginal suppositories like prasterone (Intrarosa), or the vaginal ring Estring.

"Vaginal estrogen is incredibly safe," Dr. Kelly Casperson told me. "There are very few people who can't be on it. The American College of Obstetricians and Gynecologists now has an online position statement saying that if you have had breast cancer or uterine cancer, vaginal estrogen is safe. I always say, check with your oncologist, especially if you're still in cancer treatment, in case you might be a very specific individual who should wait for some reason. But the quality of life that estrogen therapy gives people can be wonderful."

Dr. Sharon Malone told me, "I think the biggest misperception out there is that women feel that getting treatment, and particularly hormone treatment, is a dangerous option. Women are always weighing pros and cons: *I feel really bad, but if I choose hormones (which are the most surefire way to feel better and more productive), I'm taking a big risk with my health.* Nothing could be further from the truth. And I think that we in medicine must own how women got that notion in their heads."

Back to the WHI study. What was never communicated: the study wasn't created to decide if hormone therapy was effective for the symptoms of menopause—we knew it was. By this point, HRT had been used to help women with menopause symptoms for fifty years! The study was intended to see if HRT was *also* beneficial in decreasing the risk of cardiovascular disease. So it was tried in women aged fifty to seventy-nine. The average age of women in the study was sixty-three, and the majority of them were not in great health to begin with.

When the WHI stopped the study in 2002, it was because they did not see the decrease in heart disease among these older women and they claimed to have found a small increase in breast cancer (though Dr. Bluming points out that it was very slight). What should have gone out to the media was this: "There's no evidence yet that older, postmenopausal women should take HRT in order to prevent heart disease."

Instead, because of botched messaging, alarm bells sounded around the world and the study's abrupt end became this blatantly incorrect message: "HRT causes breast cancer! Every single woman on earth should throw away her pills immediately!"

"That was basically game, set, match, in terms of the case made to women for just using hormones in general," Dr. Malone told me. "And the unfortunate thing is that not only did it stop that study, but it almost singlehandedly shut down research in menopause around the world for over two decades."

Investigators involved in the WHI study have since walked back virtually all of their original scary findings—with no press conference to inform us women and our doctors. "And so here we are, more than twenty years later, still trying to fight back this notion that estrogen causes breast cancer. It does not," said Dr. Malone.

So after the WHI study and the chaos left in its wake, medicine essentially abandoned women in menopause. I can't stop thinking of the millions of women suffering with menopause, given no relief even though there is a viable option with a ton of research behind it! How much does a woman *really* need to suffer? As it turns out, maybe not as much as she thinks she does. Hormone therapy can make a huge difference.

And yet, I know a lot of women with such an aversion to pharmaceutical companies that they prefer toughing out a headache to taking an aspirin. I respect that position, just as I do the alternative. Do what you need!

In terms of non-hormonal treatments, hot-flash-combating drug Veozah is still pretty new as of this writing, and it's expensive, but it's being prescribed now, especially for women who prefer not to take hormones. I'd personally rather see more data on it, but I'm happy that new medications are being developed in response to women speaking up and identifying a need. Many doctors say if you are 100 percent ruling out HRT for treating symptoms, the next best thing is exercise, for all the usual reasons: strength, cognitive improvement, cardio/heart health, mood, sleep, and so on.

My friend said an endocrinologist told her: "This is not sexy, but you need to sleep, you need to drink less, you need to eat more protein, you need to build muscle—the old-fashioned stuff."

That kind of regimen can go a long way toward addressing concerns of women in menopause. I am just keen for women not to minimize their suffering or cut themselves off from any possible forms of relief because of misinformation.

The most important thing is to find a doctor who will have an open conversation with you about treatments for menopause symptoms and won't dismiss your individual concerns or your preferences. Dr. Rocio Salas-Whalen says, "Your best bet is to ask before you make an appointment with your doctor if they prescribe HRT. Don't assume a doctor will, regardless of their specialty."

I personally have learned so much from the conferences that are going on around the country. I've cohosted several with my friend

Alisa Volkman's group The Swell, a community and learning platform that helps women navigate the second half of their lives.

"If your doctor is gatekeeping and telling you what you can and cannot have, that's a problem," said Dr. Malone. "I mean, doctors prescribe medications every day that are far riskier, and that have never even been studied in women, without a moment's hesitation. Yet, when it comes to hormones, women are warned and even blocked from receiving the medications that will treat their symptoms and could quite possibly even save their lives. This paternalistic view about how we view women and women's health has got to go. No doctor should ever say to a grown woman: '*No, no, dear, you can't have that.*'"

I've been persuaded that HRT is actually a huge gift to many of us who otherwise would spend years in discomfort.

One woman I know who went into menopause at forty-seven told me, "I didn't feel like myself at all. I was really stressed and I couldn't sleep at night. I was getting hot flashes, and I felt exhausted and isolated and couldn't get support. Finally, I requested a woman doctor over the age of fifty. I wanted to speak to someone who understood it from experience. The doctor did understand, and she was so lovely that I started crying in her office. I started HRT and began to come back to myself."

Dr. Malone again: "If hormone therapy did nothing other than improve the quality of your life, that would be good enough, but there are actually long-term health benefits such as decreased risk of type 2 diabetes, a decrease in hip fractures, and a decrease in hospitalizations for urinary tract infections in the elderly. And for women who take estrogen only? Here's the showstopper! Their risk of developing breast cancer and risk of *dying* from breast cancer *decreased*. Not only that, but long-term studies show that women who use hormones have an increase in life expectancy. Where was the press conference for that? And that's what I keep saying, 'Well, why didn't anyone come back and correct the record?' We're doing that now: For women who are symptomatic in perimenopause or after menopause, in the postmenopausal years, the most effective treatment for symptoms is hormone therapy. Period, end of sentence."

Women, of course, should make their own choices. Plenty of women may choose not to take hormone therapy. However, you should make that decision based on your own symptoms and medical and family history.

One story that stuck with me came from Dr. Avrum Bluming, the medical oncologist, who had a personal connection to breast cancer that I found moving:

"My wife, Martha, was diagnosed with breast cancer at age forty-five. She was still very much premenopausal, and I had to treat her. It looked like chemotherapy would give her the best chance of cure. And I gave her chemotherapy. It induced medical menopause with all of the symptoms of that kind of acute menopause.

"She had the hot flushes, she had the insomnia, she had joint pain. And then she found that when she was reading a book, she couldn't remember what she had read three pages back, and that was intolerable. Martha is a huge reader and student and scholar. Because of that, I started getting very interested in the field. In the course of cancer treatment, I was responsible for inducing menopause in many women. I thought symptoms lasted one or two years. Then I learned that they last a median of 7.4 years [in white women], a little less in Asian women, more in Black and Hispanic women, and that symptoms can be truly debilitating."

And that was when he did the work to understand hormone therapy and how it could benefit women like Martha, whose brain fog rapidly cleared once she began estrogen.

Many physicians advise against giving HRT to survivors of "hormone receptor-positive" breast cancer, as this type of cancer is believed to be "fed" by hormones. But according to Dr. Bluming there is not universal consensus here either. It's worth speaking with your doctor about your options for relief even in these cases. Endocrinologist Dr. Rocio Salas-Whalen agrees: "For some women with severe symptoms, quality of present life may weigh heavier than the possibility of BRCA recurrence—such patients deserve a conversation."

The point is: HRT is much safer than we've been led to believe. It's a viable and excellent option for many women. If you decide it's right for you, the question then becomes how to take it, which we'll cover more in the next chapter. But the good news is that we have a much more nuanced approach to HRT now than we ever had before.

"Before the Women's Health Initiative study, it was thought that hormone therapy was appropriate for all women," Dr. Manson said. "After, it was thought to be appropriate for no women. Now the pendulum has landed in a reasonable place. What we learned from the WHI is that hormone therapy really should not be used for the express purpose of trying to prevent heart disease, stroke, dementia, other chronic diseases in women. But if a woman is suffering with menopause symptoms, then the benefits of treatment will likely outweigh risks. All medications have risks, and all medications involve trade-offs. For most women with moderate-to-severe symptoms in early menopause, those small risks would be more than offset by the benefits in symptom reduction and improved quality of life."

However, Dr. Mary Claire Haver, author of *The New Menopause* (and the foreword to this book) emphasizes that menopausal hormone therapy can be preventative for so many serious health issues. New research is finding that women on HRT have lower incidences of tinnitus, vertigo, frozen shoulder, palpitations, joint pain, and more. The debate continues among doctors about whether hormone therapy is merely helpful for addressing symptoms or has additional benefits beyond symptom relief.

Again, it's not that the original WHI study results were incorrect but that they were sensationalized and presented without context: the study participants were older and at higher risk for adverse events.

I wasn't alone in breathing a huge sigh of relief when *The New*

York Times published a great, viral piece by Susan Dominus in 2023: "Women Have Been Misled About Menopause: Hot Flashes, Sleeplessness, Pain During Sex: For Some of Menopause's Worst Symptoms, There's an Established Treatment. Why Aren't More Women Offered It?"

Finally, I thought.

Things They Really Should Tell Us About Hormones

- Menopause involves changes in levels of various hormones. Many symptoms of menopause are linked to the decline of estrogen, which is connected to everything from internal heat regulation to vaginal moisture to mood.

- The idea that HRT gives women breast cancer was widely popularized by the Women's Health Initiative study more than two decades ago, which actually wasn't about whether hormones helped women treat symptoms or improve quality of life during menopause, but rather whether HRT had potential benefits for cardiovascular health and prevention of chronic disease in older women.

- Estrogen-only therapy can reduce the chance of breast cancer in women without a uterus.

- Among the health benefits of hormone therapy: reduction in hot flashes, night sweats, and other menopausal symptoms; a decrease in the risk of type 2 diabetes; a decrease in the risk of osteoporosis (bone weakening) and hip fracture; and more.

- Many doctors are also still misinformed about hormones because the panic over the WHI study froze research and training. You may need to look for a doctor who's educated in menopause medicine.

CHAPTER SEVEN

IF I WANT TO TAKE HORMONES, HOW DO I DO IT?

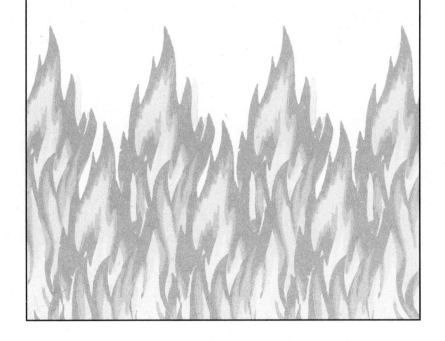

M any women I know are flummoxed by all the different options for hormones, not to mention delivery methods, and by how fast opinions seem to be evolving. "When I got out of my fourteen-year marriage, one of my friends told me that there has been a trend change, and I needed to remove all pubic hair," one friend told me. "When it comes to HRT, I feel like this is happening again!"

Once you decide you want to try hormone therapy, there are just so many options. Estrogen and/or progesterone and/or testosterone? If you are advised to take progesterone, you might be given the option to take it as a pill, a cream, an IUD, or an implanted pellet, and if you opt for a pill, you might take it every day, or for twelve consecutive days out of the month. And then there are the surprising warnings, like not to take your HRT with grapefruit juice (because it affects an enzyme that helps to metabolize medication). The lack of alignment within the medical community on the best form of delivery could be part of what's led to so much confusion among women looking for a definitive answer about what's best for them.

When I asked friends about what they'd tried, the answers were all over the place, though most of those I asked were very happy with whatever version of hormone therapy they'd ultimately settled on, praising everything from their vaginal wall's enhanced elasticity, which reduced incontinence, to the abatement of their mood swings and better sleep because of the absence of night sweats.

One said: "For me, the best thing about HRT is not so much the lubrication of my once again plumped-up parts, but the much better continence that comes with it (I have four children). Sadly, however, there is nothing sexy about the trial and error that comes with hormone therapy, nothing sexy at all. We used to laugh at how making love to me was a bit like removing the sticky bar code from the peach before consuming. You could gauge my libido by the number of glue rings patterned around my belly and hips. I remember one postcoital experience seeing the estrogen patch that had been stuck near my groin hanging off the trail of hair leading up to my husband's belly button. Getting that glue off your body requires so many showers and so much rubbing. Hardly makes you feel 'like a natural woman.'" I, of course, could relate to that story! (See Chapter 3.)

A second friend said: "I took the estradiol gel, which you put on the inside of your thigh, along with a progesterone pill. But even with insurance, the gel cost me $450 for a three-month supply. So then I got a patch. You wear the patch on your hip or abdomen and then you take the same progesterone pill. Then I went to another endocrinologist, who suggested I try a different form of progesterone because the synthetic form was thought to be provoking anxiety. From there I switched to a combination estrogen-progesterone pill."

(A note on prescription medication costs and insurance coverage: doctors I spoke with said these are highly variable. Dr. Kelly Casperson recommends comparison shopping with the help of a prescription app like Cost Plus Drugs, Amazon Pharmacy, or GoodRx. She said when picking up progesterone she was quoted $210 out of pocket or $103 to be billed to insurance, but she knew to look it up on GoodRx, so she was able to say, "I want the thirty-two-dollar price," and that's what she paid.)

Another woman told me: "It took me years to find the pill that worked best for me. At last, I could get rid of my symptoms. I'll be on my pill for as long as I can."

And finally, one woman said, "I grew up with severe endometriosis, which required two surgeries, one in my late twenties and the second in my early thirties. It was then that my body had, unbeknownst to me, stopped ovulating. Sadly, it took several years for me to realize it. My gyno, along with the normal gyno stuff, was an antiaging guru who dabbled in fen-phen lollipops, human growth hormone, and more. I arrived in his office one day, and he said to me, 'I can see the dark cloud above you.'"

After a lot of shame and confusion, she found a less woo-woo menopause specialist who put her on estrogen. "It was glorious. I immediately saw an improvement. But sadly, my inconsistent behavior kicked in, and I would go too long without changing the patch or I would put one on and forget to take the other off . . . My lower abdomen looked like one giant skin graft due to me sticking them anywhere and everywhere! My doctor finally gave me the pellet, a little thing that goes under the skin once every four months with both estrogen and testosterone in it. Where had this been all my life?" Cut to a few months later, she ran into complications with the pellet, and she's now switching to a vaginal ring.

Our menopause-treatment conversations now mirror the way we talked twenty years ago about sleep-training, breastfeeding, and potty training our kids. There's just as much scrambling for solutions and trading of suggestions. And, just as back in those days, when a good pediatrician or nursery school teacher could put me on a path that felt promising, I had confidence in my doctor when he said, "You might want to try HRT." When I was forty-two, he put me on an FDA-approved estrogen spray called Evamist, which you spritz on your arm.

I had lunch with a friend after my appointment. I whispered to her that I'd just been given *hormones*. I pulled the bottle out of my bag and stealthily showed it to her.

"Oh, I've been on that for years!" she said and teased me for being so shy.

Gradually, I came to accept that I was in a place in my life where I was on hormones. It helped a lot that I had faith in my doctor. He was savvy about the research. He told me the full story of HRT risks and benefits. He asked all the right questions. He also knew my medical history, but we talked through it all over again. He listened carefully to my symptoms. It didn't hurt that I had a crush on him. (Isn't it an amazing coincidence, how the most attractive men are also the best listeners?)

Going on hormone therapy wasn't a silver bullet for every last issue I had, but it did provide instant, massive relief. I no longer woke up sweating in the middle of the night, convinced my blankets were trying to kill me. But I soon realized I was on too low a dose to prevent emotional volatility. So many things that I ordinarily wouldn't have reacted to felt worthy of a major fight. And so, in my mid- to late forties, I upped the dosage and went from using hormones in spray form to wearing the lowest-dose patch. My moods leveled out.

The first year you're on hormones is likely to be a time of experimentation. I started at a quarter of a patch and went to half very quickly. I think it wasn't that long before I got to a full patch, but then I moved to a pill, then I moved back to patches, and now I'm on gel, and I'm sticking to it (ha). I even tried the ring for a while, which was nice because I didn't have to think about the constant applying, and because it offers both systemic and local protection—but it's pricey, and insurance won't cover it.

Unlike some people I know, I don't find the gel messy. I save it for after the shower and spend a few minutes naked before getting dressed. Plus, I use a little estrogen cream in, on, and around the vag, which keeps it plump and helps prevent UTIs. I've trusted my doctor and stayed on each method as long as I was told to. And the dosage has been adjusted several times.

Obviously, all of these decisions will be made with the guidance of a doctor, who will help you keep adjusting until you find the right delivery method and dosage.

"If you're looking for hormone therapy, you should know there are two general types of estrogen," Dr. Jen Gunter told me. "One is estradiol, which is the hormone that, for all intents and purposes, is just like what's made by your ovaries. It's semi-synthetic, meaning it is made in a lab from something found in nature. Typically, that is what's used as first-line therapy. Although some people do better with the other form, Premarin, which is extracted from the urine of pregnant horses. Those are the two formulations that we use commonly, and both have advantages and disadvantages depending on your specific needs." (A note on the term "bioidentical": it means that the molecular structure is the same as the estrogen made by your ovaries.)

The horse urine option threw me the first time I heard about it, though the name wasn't hiding anything: Premarin, from "**preg-nant mare urine.**" This version of HRT is extremely common, with something like nine million women taking it each year. It's been prescribed since 1942 and became especially common in the 1960s, thanks to gynecologist Robert Wilson's wacky but popular 1966 book *Feminine Forever*. He called menopause "a serious, painful, and often crippling disease" and said that without treatment a menopausal woman in charge might turn a workweek into "a futile, inefficient round of violent ups and downs, adult tantrums, and pointless chicanery."

Talk about paternalistic! Infuriating!

Opinions differ about how long to stay on HRT, but my current doctor is nearly seventy years old and says that she herself will never stop using it. She tells me that the benefits of estrogen can be significant even for older women—improving bone density, for starters—and that she sees any risks as negligible by comparison. Most doctors whom I've talked to say that there's a natural window of opportunity for women, around the time of menopause, where there is a clear benefit and low risk. Beyond that time frame, some experts think it makes sense to stop, and others, like my doctor, believe in staying on it indefinitely. She puts estrogen gel on her neck, and she looks great.

The problem is often that when you're on HRT and no longer having symptoms, you don't know if you still need it. Generally, doctors I've spoken to suggest going on it for a couple of years and then doing an annual assessment, asking yourself questions about how you're feeling. (Another consideration: when you stop estrogen therapy you will lose bone density, which could increase your risk of osteoporosis and fractures.) Meanwhile, urologist Dr. Rachel Rubin tells her patients that vaginal hormones may be taken "'til death do you part."

Of course, because of the reaction to the Women's Health Initiative study (discussed in the previous chapter), a whole generation of doctors are not receiving any clinically significant training in menopause and are not comfortable prescribing hormone therapy. And so the market has come to be flooded with people selling all kinds of snake oil.

Dr. Jen Gunter has done much to bring science to bear on various myths concerning menopause, like the idea that we need compounded hormones instead of the hormones traditionally prescribed.

"'Synthetic' doesn't mean bad," Dr. Gunter said, "In fact, sometimes synthetic is better. Maybe the synthetics have less troublesome side effects, or more benefit. We would never have had the birth control pill without synthetic hormones."

She added that *compounded* hormones are more unpredictable in the dosage you're getting than traditional hormone therapy from a pharmaceutical company, and they are not approved by the FDA.

Dr. Stacy Lindau said that when in doubt about hormones or supplements, it's usually good to check out Menopause Society guidelines, because the society's members are the people spending the most time looking carefully at these issues. "I wish that we could rely on compounded regimens because some people really prefer them," she said. "We need to hear women when they say they feel better about compounded hormones and understand why. It just points out that there's a gap in terms of options we're providing for women. Why would people be opting for compounded therapies or off-label therapies or understudied therapies? What do those choices say about women's trust in science and the medical establishment, and what do we learn from that to do better? We need to hear women who are making those choices. My concern is, and I have the same concern for vitamins and supplements, do I really know what I'm putting in my body and am I better off with the uncertain thing I'm putting in my body or without it?"

To me, these seem like good questions to ask. If a woman is taking something unproven, why? Is it because she's had experiences, and I've had plenty myself, of being talked down to by the same doctors who are then dismissing her preferences? And then can we ask ourselves if we're able to make decisions based on the science without being too swayed by our understandable mistrust of authority figures?

I find it notable that as more women have begun taking hormone therapy, there have been shortages. Recently, I was down to my last three progesterone pills and was told they were on back order for weeks. The distress that came over me! I was afraid I was in for weeks of sleepless nights. But then I was comforted by the notion that for the world this was good news—finally women are taking their health into their own hands and no longer scared of using HRT! This is a massive tidal change for good. And in the end—praise be!—I managed to get my hands on some pills after a wild goose chase to various pharmacies.

There was recently a patch shortage in Australia, and one friend of mine almost had a fight with a pharmacist when she was told about it. She said the other delivery methods haven't been as good for her: "I'm not in love with the gel. It has an alcohol base that reminds me of Covid hand sanitizer, and putting it on every day is just one more thing to remember and one more decision to make (right or left arm). Then I have to remember to take the pill that comes with it. Yes, in the same box, but still one more thing in a different hole."

My friend Rebecca told me a story that sums up the bewilderment the complicated menu of hormone options can cause. "I'm using the gel now after years of the patch and then three years of the estradiol pill. My doctor said the pill version can cause blood clots, especially when flying." (It's true—estrogen makes blood "stickier," and so slightly more likely to form clots.) "The gel is messy and takes ages to dry but it's safer. Because I have a major fear of flying, I was so high on a gummy and a Valium on a flight that I smeared the gel all over my arms and passed out on the seat with the bottle on my lap, like an estrogen addict. No dignity in old age."

She's right that figuring out your perfect recipe for HRT can seem to involve as much trial and error as perfecting a soufflé. But for me the effort has been more than worth it.

Things They Really Should Tell Us About How to Take Hormones

- There are a number of delivery methods (pill, patch, gel, spray, pellets—though pellets are not FDA approved—or a vaginal ring) and dosages. Work with your doctor to figure out which work best for you. Realize it might take a few months to get everything sorted out and for you find the right fit.

- Other than Premarin, all prescribed estrogens are "synthetic." That just means that they're made in a lab. The term "bioidentical" just means that the molecular structure is the same as the estrogen made by your ovaries. Contrast this with the nonbioidentical estrogen in birth control pills, ethinyl estradiol, which is safe and effective but has a different mission—to suppress ovaries, provide birth control, and control cycles.

- There are multiple formulations of estrogen—estradiol is identical to what our ovaries make, and it's the most commonly prescribed. Other options are available if needed. Your doctor will discuss what makes sense for you and whether or not you need to add in progesterone, which is given to protect the uterine lining. If you've had a hysterectomy, you can take estrogen alone.

- As with any medications, there are risks with HRT, particularly blood clots with the pill form because systemic estrogen can make blood "stickier." It's important to discuss risks with your doctor.

CHAPTER EIGHT

TELL ME AGAIN

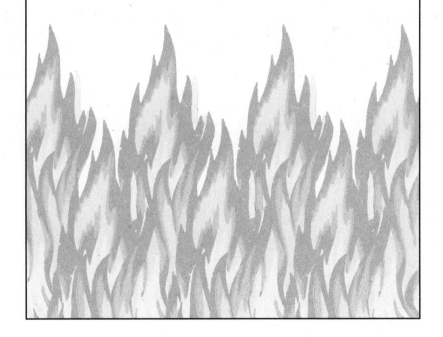

Over dinner with a friend I hadn't seen in a while, she leaned over and said she had something terrible to confess. Before I had time to imagine what horrible thing she had to tell me she said: "I lost my bike."

I was about to laugh, but then I saw her eyes fill with tears.

She continued: "I went to a meeting downtown, and when I came out, I couldn't remember where I'd parked my bike. I looked for hours. And then the next day, I kept going back to look, and I couldn't find it."

"Surely it was stolen!" I said.

"No," she said, "I just couldn't remember where it was."

Two days later, she found her bike chained up a few blocks from the meeting near a store she'd stopped into. She'd kept the episode from her family because she was so embarrassed. Her husband and children had often teased her about her forgetfulness, and she knew they'd make fun of her for losing the bike.

"What should I do?" she asked me.

"Well, for starters, surely your family should be kinder to you!" I said.

When I have these moments of forgetfulness, Billy always says, "It's no wonder. You're spinning so many plates."

After all, who among us hasn't forgotten where we parked our car or where we left our keys? One friend of mine recalls a time when she took her child on a college tour and then spent a full hour bickering with him about his plan to bring his girlfriend to college while they wandered through every parking lot on campus looking for her car.

Not long ago, I was at the airport heading to the Golden Globes. I was texting away with my friends and got so consumed that I missed the boarding call for my flight. By the time I looked up, they'd closed the door, and even though the plane sat at the gate for another forty-five minutes, they wouldn't let me on. I was so mad at myself for spacing out. The next available flight was packed, so I had to sit with my gown on my lap the whole way, because there was no luggage space left.

So I knew what my bike friend was talking about! But looking back, I realized that we'd had trouble scheduling the dinner. She had laughed off her calendar confusion as ditziness, but in general she seemed to vacillate between minimizing her cognitive problems—"I'm just a little forgetful sometimes"—and wondering if she might be losing her mind.

Again, I'm no stranger to the humiliation caused by memory loss. How much anxiety that has brought me over the years! Surely we've all played rounds of "Oh, look! It's that person in the movie who is in that other movie with so-and-so!" But I've also had moments in press junkets where I forgot not only names of actors I'd worked with for months but even the name of the actual movie! When I feel that blankness coming, I'm flooded with anxiety. I resort to saying "thingy" as a placeholder for a word or name I can't remember.

It happened to me the other day when I was at dinner with Ryan Murphy. I said, "I've been in London doing the Lena Dunham show."

Oh no, I thought. *He's going to ask me what it's called. What was it called? I had the best time! She's so fantastic. What was written on the call sheet? Was it two words? Ugh! Okay, wait, maybe he won't ask me. I'll take a sip of water and change the subject and—*

"What's it called?" he said.

Cue *blind panic.*

"Thingy . . ."

I'd literally *just* left the set of *Too Much.* Why and how could this happen? I think it was the recall of the previous times its happened. Something takes over, that inner voice creeping in . . . "You are going to forget . . . you are such an idiot, here it comes and . . ." BOOM! The name is gone—only to return the precise moment I give up, so that I blurt it out half an hour later when we are deep into another conversation.

At a press event with my costars on *Feud: Capote vs. The Swans* we were asked, "When you think about the distance that women have traversed since those days when the most privileged women of society were thinking about what they were going to wear to the Black and White Ball, would you choose that kind of privilege if you could?"

"Well, speaking for myself, this is the greatest role I've had for quite a few years," I began. "I'm really proud of the piece of work, and it's landing with audiences." *Strong start, doing great.* "I think there are parallels to be drawn. We're still fighting for relevance, I suppose, like these women were, but I think that comes whether you're male and female, that comes from midlife." *Uh, where are we going now?* "There's not so much judgment, we're not judging ourselves. At this point in time, we're learning to love because we're living longer, I think, optimizing our health so that we can enjoy this time being in the middle of our lives . . ."

At this point I noticed the other Swans looking at me quizzically. With my eyes, I tried to signal to them: *Well, sorry! There I went! Bit of a tangent there.*

What I've tried to do in these situations is to own it. The way I used to handle such moments was to blush and wish the earth would open up and swallow me whole. Now I just try to call out what's happening: "I've been doing a lot of menopause lectures. My brain got confused for a second about where I was. Please forgive me and let's get back on track!" People relax. Everyone understands that feeling.

I don't want to minimize it, though. Memory loss is a real peril of middle age. And whether it's related to brain fog caused by brain changes or caused by sleep loss, which is also so common at this age, the effect is the same. Without your memory, you can start to feel like a shell of yourself. You wonder who you are. Not only do you not know how to function in the new version of yourself, but you are also afraid that the self you've been for your whole life is never coming back.

I suggested that my friend might go to the doctor to rule out something more serious, though that was extremely unlikely. This sort of forgetfulness is something so many women I know contend with. One told me that she and a friend once spent an entire car trip trying to recall the book title *The Bonfire of the Vanities*.

The person who's most helped me to understand the menopausal brain is Dr. Lisa Mosconi, a neuroscientist, educator, and author known for her books *The Menopause Brain* and *The XX Brain*. She is also the director of the Women's Brain Initiative and director of the Alzheimer's Prevention Clinic, both at Weill Cornell Medicine, where she is an associate professor of neuroscience in neurology and radiology.

Dr. Mosconi, who grew up in Florence, Italy, got interested in the field because she has a family history of Alzheimer's disease. Her grandmother was one of four siblings, three sisters and one brother, and all three sisters developed dementia or Alzheimer's disease and died of it. The brother was spared, even though they all lived to the same age. There was little support in the Italian healthcare system for dementia prevention. To figure out a way to help herself and others, Lisa got a dual PhD in neuroscience and nuclear medicine, the latter so she could do radiology for prevention.

"During my studies, I went to my PhD mentor and said, 'Does it matter if you're a woman or a man when it comes to Alzheimer's disease?'" she told me. "The answer was, 'Sort of.' Because Alzheimer's is a disease of old age, and women tend to live longer than men, unfortunately, more women than men end up developing it. But what we've learned is that it's a disease that starts in midlife, with symptoms that become evident in old age."

Certainly, I know a lot of women who feel like menopause changed their brains. One told me she felt there was a connection between her memory issues and her menopausal mood swings: "I would go from crying at the sight of a squirrel eating a nut to having a full sweat mustache while standing in front of the freezer, forgetting why I opened it in the first place. The long pauses got longer. The blank stares alarmed those who knew me. Some joked that I was having a stroke, and honestly, I thought at times I was because I couldn't remember the smallest detail, and I thought staring at nothing would bring it back into my head. I kept calling people and then forgetting why, so I'd hang up and text them, 'Sorry, pocket dial!'" This is the kind of strategy I need!

For years, when my kids misbehaved, I would confiscate something from them, like a toy or a Nintendo. I couldn't put the confiscated objects in the same place because my kids would find the hiding places, so I had to hide things in more obscure places each time. Then, when it was time to give the toy back, I often couldn't remember where it was. I'd go on endless searches and then say, "I'm adding a day until you get it back!" My kids started to catch on. They began to call me out for not remembering. We couldn't find the older one's Nintendo for months.

When I tried to tell a friend about how bad my memory had gotten, she said, "No! You memorize lines every day!"

Yes, but every actor has had the nightmare of being naked onstage, having forgotten all her lines. And memorizing lines is focused work and short term. We can all keep track of things for a little while, but will I remember a single one of those lines in a month? No way. Not to mention, we're saying lines of dialogue that are someone else's. When we're saying dialogue, we don't have to fear the same judgment about saying the wrong thingy.

Dr. Mosconi hears memory-loss stories a lot, and she is eager for more people to be aware of the connection between memory loss and our hormones: "Nobody had told me in school that menopause had an impact on the brain. Now menopause is at the heart of pretty much all the research that we're doing."

The link makes intuitive sense. When you think about what happens to women throughout the course of their reproductive lives—PMS, postpartum depression, mood disturbances during perimenopause—surely, it's all the same hormones?

"I find it so aggravating that the medical field does not believe in sex differences," said Dr. Mosconi. "We call it 'bikini medicine,' which basically says that what makes a woman a woman—from a medical perspective—are those body parts that can be covered by a bikini. Your reproductive organs and nothing more. So medical professionals, forever, have really treated and diagnosed women and men the same, except for those different body parts. And unfortunately there's this misconception in neuroscience that hormones don't matter, that the brains of men and women should be under the same microscope."

In studying women's health, I've learned that women were typically not even used in trials sponsored by the National Institutes of Health until Congress passed a law requiring their inclusion—in 1993! But that was thirty years ago. Hasn't science grown more curious about women since then? Why has there still been so little research into menopause and the brain?

"The answer is that there's no money in it," says Dr. Mosconi. "And if you're a scientist, you need to pay the bills. During the last reporting period, the National Institutes of Health spent $45 billion of our taxpayer money funding research. Women make up 51 percent of the population, but research into health concerns primarily impacting them only got about 10 percent of that money. . . . So a lot of areas in women's health go unfunded, menopause being chief among them. We deserve so much more."

Women are two-thirds of dementia patients. Some of the reason for that can be attributed to women living longer, but that's not the whole story. Something about women makes them more susceptible to Alzheimer's. But what?

Dr. Mosconi decided to do brain scans of women before and after menopause. What she saw impressed her deeply. As women aged, the activity in the frontal cortex (the part of your brain in charge of thinking and reasoning) as well as the cingulate cortex (which handles remembering things you've done) and temporal cortex (in charge of overall memory and function) dropped by about 30 percent on average.

Some women don't show these changes. The drop could be very mild. But some show it severely.

One woman I know said, "I used to have an excellent memory—like a weird, almost photographic memory. Nothing useful, but I'd remember everyone's birthdays, and could rattle off all the presidents in ten seconds. That was a good party trick. But now I can't remember what I had for dinner yesterday. I can't remember what the Wordle was. And I don't know if it's just because of brain fog or because at this point in my life I have so much in my head that I actually need to care about that I can't keep track of the minutiae anymore."

She worries about dementia because her grandmother had it, so she takes "brain health" supplements even though there's no evidence that people without nutritional deficiency benefit from them.

Dr. Mosconi said, "A lot of women come to us because they're concerned that they can't function the way they used to and assume it's a sign of early dementia, so we have to do very thorough examinations—lots of lab work, MRIs, and PET scans—to be able to tell with certainty whether it's menopause or not."

And if it's menopause, what can be done?

Dr. Mosconi's team just completed the largest-ever examination of the effect of hormone therapy on Alzheimer's disease and dementia, with more than six million women from all over the world involved.

"If you look at all the data together, estrogen-only therapy started in midlife was associated with more than a 30 percent reduced risk of Alzheimer's disease in late life. Now, that's good news. If you start taking estrogen-only therapy more than ten years after the last menstrual period, the effect is neutral. Doesn't harm you, doesn't protect you. The estrogen-progesterone combination taken in midlife was also associated with a mild risk reduction, about 23 percent lower risk."

The news for people like me, who went into early menopause, is dramatic, according to Mosconi: "If you enter menopause before the age of forty-five, that in and of itself is a risk factor for developing Alzheimer's." Yikes! For those of us in early menopause, she says hormone therapy could be one way to lower that risk.

Phew! I did something right (fingers crossed).

But regardless of when we start menopause, hormone therapy doesn't offer full protection. So what else can women do?

"Start prevention as soon as you can," says Dr. Mosconi. "There are quite a few things that can improve brain health at any age. They take discipline. Number one is getting regular medical check-ups. We need to manage conditions that are known to increase the risk of Alzheimer's disease: metabolic disorders like diabetes, insulin resistance, prediabetes, and obesity, as well as cardiovascular disease. High blood pressure needs to get managed. High cholesterol needs to get managed. High triglycerides need to get managed. Managing thyroid disease is very important, too. Menopause, I think, should become part of the neurological workup to prevent dementia."

She also recommends a good diet involving more plants, as they can reduce oxidative stress inside the brain. Also, of course, exercise. "We don't move nearly enough as a population. Many of us sit a lot, but it's really important to find ways to move our bodies."

Then she said one thing that surprised me: "Hygiene is another factor. Brushing your teeth is really important because the oral and gut microbiomes impact your brain health. If you have dysbiosis (where your microbiome is out of whack), you may get brain fog or mental fatigue. Make sure to floss, too." I've always been so lazy about flossing. Since I heard that the germs in our mouths affect our gut microbiome, I have definitely upped my game!

So gut health and brain health are linked because of the microbiome, and heart health is also brain health. It's all connected! The same things that you would do to minimize your risk of cardiovascular disease are the behaviors and lifestyle modifications you need to make to reduce your risk for Alzheimer's. There can also be a genetic component to your risk for developing Alzheimer's. It's good to rule all that out.

And remember: the forgetfulness so many of us experience around this age could be a sign of hormonal fluctuation that causes real changes to how our brains work. These are changes we can treat or mitigate with HRT and lifestyle changes.

My bike friend finally went to the doctor. Her MRI came back clear, so her brain fog is likely menopause related. She's going to explore HRT. Meanwhile, I encouraged her to sit her family down and tell them to stop adding to her stress! Whatever is going on, it's something that requires loving attention, not jokes.

Things They Really Should Tell Us About Brain Health

- Brain fog—like hot flashes—can be a symptom of menopause. Lab work, MRIs, and PET scans can help determine whether it is indicative of a dementia-related issue. If it's menopause related, HRT can help.

- New and updated studies have shown that the use of estrogen in midlife can reduce the risk of developing Alzheimer's disease. This is particularly true for those in early menopause.

- Not to be too woo-woo, but meditation and breathwork can help with anxiety, and calming down can help us remember things.

- Much of the same work you do to prevent cardiovascular issues (maintaining a diet full of plant-based foods, getting regular exercise) can also help with brain issues. Take care of your metabolic health.

- Tell the people around you to be gentle with you.

CHAPTER NINE

DRYING UP

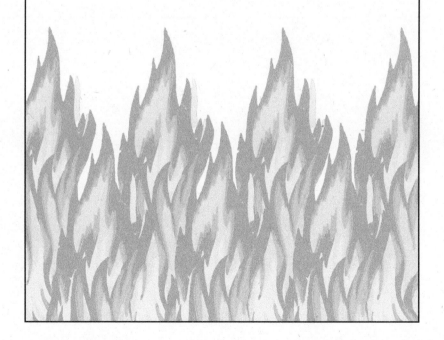

H ere is a real conversation a friend of mine had with her boyfriend:

HER: Honey, I want to do something with my face. I want to get my neck done. I want to get rid of my double chin.

HIM: No! You're beautiful the way you are! You've earned your wrinkles! They're part of what I love about you! Haven't you always said you wanted to age naturally?

HER: Well, Marie Kondo was all about precision and spotlessness until she had kids. People's priorities change. When I look in the mirror all I see are these horrible jowls. I don't want to look like a different person. I just want to look a little bit less tired.

HIM: What if you look different? It would be like being with someone else.

HER: No, it will still be me.

He looked at his girlfriend in a long, serious way. She felt the compassion and empathy. She felt seen and heard. How lucky she was to have found a man who loved her, wrinkles and all. Finally, he sighed.

HIM: Okay. And if you're already there, can you throw in some tits as well?

I'm pretty sure that after I went on and on about facelifts, I—I mean, my friend!—deserved that comment, as well as what followed, when the boyfriend threatened to have a facelift himself. That was when I knew that it was time to change the subject.

Women all have their own calculations about the degree to which they want to stay natural as they age or if they want to go all in on interventions. Some do nothing, or just use daily sunscreen for prevention. Others, especially those who can afford it, have their cosmetic dermatologists on speed dial or have had minimal to multiple surgeries. Where you fall on the continuum has everything to do with your personal taste, your level of disposable income, and how much societal pressure you've been subjected to about looking young.

In my forties, I started having itchy, irritable skin. I told everyone, "I'm on camera, and I can't stop scratching my face! What do I do?" I tried cortisone ointment, and it would help in the short term, but it was just a temporary fix. (Long-term use is associated with various side effects, including adrenal gland problems and thinning of the skin.) I didn't know that itchy skin was linked to menopause, whereas I now know that the loss of estrogen causes dehydration through our entire bodies.

Looking for products that would treat my easily inflamed skin, I reached out to my girlfriends who had created a retail business called Onda Beauty, which sells entirely clean, natural products. They gave me some things that helped instantly. My skin did so well with those gentler ingredients. Then I started looking more closely at the brands I'd been using. I noticed quite harsh ingredients that were no longer working for me as well as overblown promises of age reversal. I couldn't help but note that these anti-wrinkle creams had marketing campaigns full of women half my age. This is when I saw that we needed more options that worked and honest guidance about what products could and couldn't do, as well as education about our profound need for moisturizing during menopause.

This is the phase of life when we're more likely to have time to invest in ourselves. We don't go to bed with our makeup on anymore. We don't just take thirty seconds to brush our teeth and then call it a night. We have patience for the extra steps that will make sure our skin feels good in the morning. And we'll treat ourselves to quality skin care rather than splurging on the trendy little black dress or a new pair of sneakers.

I thought, *What if there was a brand geared toward this age that had products for all parts of our bodies, addressing the whole spectrum of symptoms?* What if there was a place to go that took all the cherry-picking out of self-care for women in midlife, the endless dance of *I've got to go to this store for my hair care, I've got to go to that health food store for my vitamins, I've got to go here for this and there for that?* What if it was all a one-stop shop, and we weren't overpromising, but we were telling you, "We see you. You are vibrant and still relevant, and we want to empower you with education and a community, as well as offer these products tailored to your needs, from scalp to vag, with very specific, targeted ingredients."

I also wanted the beauty line to be fun, sexy, irreverent, and bold, and to make it clear to women my age: This is not the end. This is not the time to pull out the knitting needles and sit in the corner. This is a time to take good care of ourselves and to embrace joy. (Though I should say that I have recently taken up knitting! But not because I'm in retirement; because it's soothing and meditative and helps me remember my lines!)

Having grown up in the United Kingdom and Australia, where it's culturally ingrained to be self-deprecating and to shrink and apologize for everything, I've always found it hard to speak up for myself. I had tremendous culture shock when I came to America. Everyone seemed so confident! But at last, even I in my chronic shyness felt compelled to do something. The only public figure I remembered talking about hormones and menopause seemed to be Suzanne Somers. She was a pioneer, a baller, way ahead of her time. She was also advocating for hormone compounds, which, by the time I came around to my own menopause experience, I had learned were not approved by the FDA.

As I've said, I did worry that publicly identifying myself with menopause would say to Hollywood that I was no longer relevant.

I'd been told by more than one person in the industry that I'd better work as much as possible, because forty is when it all dries up,
pardon the pun. But I wanted to figure out a way to connect menopausal women and to feel less alone myself.

After starting to talk about my own experience, I was struck by
the extent of women's suffering and their loneliness, as well as their
need to feel seen. On more than a few occasions, I've had women
come up to me with tears in their eyes, ready to share their stories
of finally being able to talk to partners or bosses about their experiences. These women are doing incredible things without much
support while juggling a lot of responsibility.

For my part, I felt like in many ways I was just getting started.
My career was thriving. I played Ann Darrow in *King Kong* at
thirty-six, just before I got that first round of bloodwork that
branded me as being in early menopause.

Jumping way forward, when Covid happened and we all got
stuck indoors, I suddenly had time to explore options for reaching
women with the same questions I had. I'd already been closely involved with Onda Beauty, but now it was my whole focus. One day
I was on a call with about fifty beauty founders, CEOs, and inves-
tors. The question arose: What do we do to help one another? I
started to wonder what else might be possible. Those calls turned
into a meeting every week for a couple of years.

I was very anxious about taking a risk on starting a business,
but I couldn't stop thinking about it. When I began blabbing on
about menopause, I knew that I was doing something risky. No
one wants to be alone on a soapbox, shouting into the void about
such a personal and frequently taboo topic. I knew that I needed
support, and I saw the potential for forging a bigger community
around this issue—but I hadn't the foggiest idea of how to begin!
And so I did what every visionary, natural-born, true leader does: I
googled "How to create a movement."

As silly as that may sound, I soon found a TED Talk by Derek
Sivers that continues to inspire me to this day. He provided an ex-

ample of how one person got a group of people to dance in a park. A person hoping to start a dance party might begin to dance uninhibitedly and look quite foolish while everyone around them mills about, hewing closely to social norms that tell us not to get our boogie on in public, no matter how fun it looks! But maybe one person sees that person dancing and gets inspired to join in. All of a sudden two people are dancing, and they look a little less foolish. That second person calls in their friends, and their friends call in their friends, and before you know it, a full-on party breaks out in the middle of a park.

In summary, to start a social movement, Sivers says that a leader needs to be willing to be ridiculous, providing simple instructions. But even more important than that leader is the brave soul who decides to heed the call of this lone nut and join in. It's only with the enthusiasm of a follower that a regular person turns into a leader. According to Sivers, the leader is the flint, the follower is the spark, and together they make a fire. Eventually, more and more people join the cause until there's no longer any risk associated with linking up and joining in. And if a cause is successful enough, the tide turns, and there's a risk of being left behind if you don't hop on.

My dream was to create a community. I thought that by sharing our stories, we could one day live in a world where we've cut away all the stigma associated with middle age, and it's the norm to be fully, authentically ourselves at every age.

Over time, those calls and the research I was doing built my confidence. No one had made a convincing case that the world *shouldn't* pay more attention to menopausal women. But how in the living hell could I get this thing going? The people I was talking to were so inspiring. I felt the urge to do something with this idea I'd had swirling around. At the beginning of the second year, I thought, *I'm going to just make a cold call and pitch this menopause company. Let's see where it goes.* I found myself on the phone with an executive at the biotech company Amyris. He said, "Ooh, I like this idea. I'm going to get you in the room with two other people here." I began to think that even though I never finished my education, I might have some business acumen after all.

I scrambled to assemble a deck with pictures that I had collected from the internet and Instagram. It was pretty good considering I pulled it together with a colleague, who is brilliant with graphic design, in fewer than twenty-four hours. Then we had that meeting, and the executive said, "Let's do this." From that first call to the launch of Stripes Beauty, it was maybe sixteen months.

I was so happy to hear that people responded as I'd hoped they would. So many women have since told me that the Stripes Beauty website is a great place to learn about menopause, as well as a place to feel seen and reflected. In this work, I've found that humor is our greatest asset, because Lord knows there's enough misery and fear out there. It's so much easier to learn things when we defuse the suffering and pain with laughter. We need to continually ask: How do we face this time of life in a way that makes it not just bearable but fun? That's how Stripes Beauty wound up offering products like the play oil Oh My Glide and the hydrating gel Vag of Honor.

But products like these (however good they are!) are no substitute for regular visits to a dermatologist. Skin-cancer checks are essential, and dermatologists may have advice on what can be done for issues like bags under your eyes or flaking skin. These doctors aren't always in-network, but I've found that it can be cheaper even to pay out of pocket for a consultation with a good dermatologist than to try a dozen different products from the drugstore or Sephora, hoping that one serum will work where the last didn't.

Doctors who knew about menopause told me that my skin's dryness was connected to my age. Cellular turnover slows down as we grow older. In our twenties, our skin regenerates on about a monthly cycle. But in our fifties, that same cycling takes more like fifty days. And without turnover, you wind up with that feeling and appearance of dullness. Retinols and exfoliants can help speed up our skin cells' turnover, but they can also be drying, so it's a tricky balance to strike. I tend to stay away from them these days, or only use them for a special occasion.

Annoyingly, our skin at this age can be both dry and acne prone because sebaceous glands are active and prevalent all over the body. (Once again, this weird mirroring of puberty and menopause!)

"Certainly during puberty, our sebaceous glands can be overactive and lead to acne—and we're not always clear of that as we age," said Dr. Dendy Engelman, a board-certified dermatologic surgeon in New York City. "The American Academy of Dermatology says that 25 percent of women in their forties are still suffering with acne. So, they've got breakouts on their faces, and they say, 'When I said I wanted to look younger, I didn't mean acne!' They may at the same time have vaginal dryness. So, it's a grand irony of how do we moisturize one area and dry out other areas where there are breakouts?"

Dermatologist Dr. Amy Wechsler told me, "Hormonal acne is typically on the lower face, chin, jawline, neck. That's because there are more testosterone receptors on the lower face."

If a woman in her forties who hasn't had a pimple in twenty years starts breaking out, she might want to explore the possibility that it's connected to hormones.

The patient would likely have blood tests and then possibly be given birth control, or an oral medication called spironolactone, which was originally created to treat high blood pressure.

Another big issue for women at this age is rosacea, a flare-up of redness on the face. "Rosacea often can flare up or can start when someone's got skin sensitivity," said Dr. Wechsler. "I talk about having sensitive skin in two ways. You can be born with sensitive skin, have it your whole life, or you can have temporarily sensitive skin that can be induced by hormonal changes, trying new products, being super stressed, not sleeping. And so menopause is just one of those upheavals that can cause sensitivity. And then sometimes one of the ways that manifests is rosacea. Others include rashes, eczema, dermatitis. Often switching to sensitive skin, fragrance-free products helps." Certainly I used to love doing all sorts of drugstore face masks, but now my skin rebels against every one of them except the gentlest.

Once a dermatologist said I should do a chemical peel. Seconds after he applied it in the procedure room, I felt my skin burning as if it were on fire. I could feel panic rising as he quickly wiped off the chemicals. He said the recovery would take five days. On day ten, Christmas Day, I sat there with a completely crusted-over face. I'm one of those people who's already slightly depressed at Christmas, and the aftereffects of the peel did not help. We always need to do research before procedures so we don't get talked into things.

On the subject of sensitivity: my friends and I love to relax over a mani-pedi, but dermatologists have told me that when it comes to nail care we might want to be more careful about where we go and what kind of manicure we get.

Dr. Wechsler said, "UV is dangerous. A gel manicure is better if you're going to wear those gloves that have the fingertips cut off, and sunscreen, but still, the nail bed is getting exposed to the ultraviolet light. I don't like that at all." For a regular manicure, she says she doesn't like cutting the cuticle. "I never let anyone touch the bottom of my cuticle. A healthy cuticle protects the nail from getting infected with fungus, yeast, and bacteria." Finally, she says it's good to look at how the salon cleans their instruments, especially for pedicures: "If someone has fungus or a wart on their foot and they put it in that water bath and you go after them, you could catch it. Most places only clean with bleach at the end of the day. And bleach is the only thing that kills all those things. A little soapy water is not going to kill the wart virus or fungi and bacteria. In my office, I see all sorts of infections in feet and sometimes hands from nail salons. If they use a disposable liner, or if you're the first client in the morning and they clean with bleach overnight, you're usually safe."

Dr. Engelman said that getting enough sleep makes a significant difference in skin issues, because deep sleep is the stage where there's a rise in human growth hormone—and HGH is also connected to healthy hair.

Hair loss surprises a lot of women at this age. I myself didn't realize that my thinning hair was a dermatological matter and not just a problem to handle at the salon.

Dr. Wechsler says that one issue she often finds connected to hair loss in middle-aged women is a low iron level: "You're losing blood every month. My gynecologist said, 'I don't like menstruating women to donate blood. You don't have enough iron.' It makes total sense, because you give a lot when you give a whole pint of blood. I mean, it's such a nice thing to do for so many reasons, but a lot of women, even without donating blood, don't have enough iron. And hair is really dependent on iron and iron stores."

I asked her about supplements, and she said yes, they work, and that sometimes even an infusion is warranted. "If someone's still bleeding and her iron is low, you can give her IV iron and then check her bloods in a month. If her levels are normal, then how often she's menstruating and how heavy the flow determines how often to check the blood going forward, every six months to a year. It's also possible to slow down or stop heavy menstruation with birth control pills or an IUD."

Hair is my Achilles' heel. I feel like it's the one thing I can never quite get right. Obviously, I've used and abused my hair on films and fashion shoots since my twenties. I've colored it, teased it, hot-ironed it, loaded it up with product—and, worst of all, pulled it freakishly tight to give myself a DIY facelift and hidden it under wigs for days at a time.

Every person in my family has thin hair, but I have less than my grandmother, than my brother, than my aunts, than my mother. My hairline continues to recede. My part opens. I've done every supplement and treatment out there, and yes, it's become somewhat of an obsession for me. In a low moment, I had PRP, injections of platelet-rich plasma commonly used for speedy injury recovery. It caused my forehead to swell up so dramatically that I had to cancel a magazine cover shoot.

What helps me most is maintaining a high-protein, high-iron diet and minimizing stress. And trying not to abuse my poor hair like I used to unless it's absolutely necessary for work. I do have good periods, but then my hair goes back to what it was—thin and thinning. I wear wigs in films, hair extensions for shoots. Recently I found a more permanent extension option that I like, a micro-beaded process, though it has to be redone every six weeks. In some ways I'm grateful because my thinning hair distracts me from my aging face!

Whenever I've seen Dr. Engelman talk at conferences, the moment she gets to thinning hair, women in the audience always turn to each other, gesture toward her shampoo-ad-worthy long, lush blond hair, and whisper, "Well, she sure doesn't have that problem!"

But Dr. Engelman says she's seen how personal hair loss can be, whether it's connected to age or to illness. "I'm a skin cancer surgeon," she told me. "In that specialty, I've had more patients cry in my exam room while talking about their hair loss than upon hearing a skin cancer diagnosis. Hair is very emotional. People don't always know if dermatologists are the right doctors to seek out about hair loss. They say, 'I don't even know if you're the right specialist. Should I be talking to my primary care doctor? My internist? My OB?' And the truth is, we are the experts on everything on the outside: hair, skin, nails. I have to tell people: 'We don't age into better hair naturally.'

"We know there's shrinking of the hair follicle and the shaft of the hair, and we lose hair density. And in women, it doesn't present as it does with men, in what they call a 'power alley,' where they have receding hairlines. Women have widening of the middle hair part. There's more scalp showing, and that can be distressing."

So what can be done about hair loss? Women I know who are worried about losing their hair take supplements like Nutrafol, Wellbel, or Vegamour. Other women I know with hair concerns take biotin gummies even if they cause GI issues, like stomach cramps, nausea, and diarrhea. I also know a lot of women who swear by "fill-in powder" that matches their hair color. Applied to the scalp, it covers up the bare skin you otherwise see among the thinning hair.

I know: another product! If your bathroom is like mine, it's full of enough little potions to make it look like a witch's pantry. I used to merely wash my face at night; now I go through an elaborate production that could be titled *Skin Care: A Play in Four Acts.*

One: cleanser. Some dermatologists recommend a "double cleanse," in which you take off your makeup (I swear by an eye makeup remover I get at Target, Bioderma H2O Micellar Water) and then use a deeper cleanser. At this age, you'll often get a recommendation for a gentle cleanser, rather than something more astringent or exfoliating, like you might have used when you were younger. Look for a cleanser that's milky, not too foamy, and can be splashed off.

Two: toner to dampen the skin and open the pores to let the moisture in. Applied with a cotton ball or sprayed and patted on with the hand.

Three: serum. This is usually lighter than a moisturizer and can address whatever you're dealing with specifically—dryness or dullness or dark spots, for example. The Stripes Beauty formulator created a special combination of ingredients for menopausal women, squalene with ectoine, for deeper hydration. One of the most common ingredients you see in serums is hyaluronic acid, which makes skin more flexible and decreases wrinkles. Another is nicotinamide, a water-soluble version of vitamin B_3, which tightens skin, making pores smaller.

Four: Daytime, moisturizer with SPF. Nighttime, night moisturizer without SPF. These products often contain retinol or retinoids, which can increase collagen production, making skin appear plumper.

And then you have the extras: eye cream, masks, and exfoliants, not to mention pricier and more extreme injectable treatments, like Botox, which relaxes muscles for a few months, getting rid of wrinkles, or collagen filler, which fills in lines. Makeup guru Bobbi

Brown told me, "I have chosen to not get injectables. It's just not my thing. But I have been leaning into lasers and all sorts of things that I think make me look better."

She uses microcurrent treatments and masks to calm down the skin or shrink pores. Laser resurfacing can be pricey, and there can be a recovery period of a few days or even a couple of weeks, during which there's significant crusting and peeling depending on how much you do at once. But it really helps with skin evenness and vibrancy. Ask your friends about recovery periods as well as your doctors!

I have done a procedure called the Morpheus8 on my neck and face in order to increase collagen production. It can hurt like hell and is expensive, but some dermatologists consider it a good idea for firming. And it had always been my philosophy that if it doesn't hurt it's probably not doing anything. Well, then I was talking to *another* dermatologist, and she said she never does that procedure because in her experience the results don't last very long. What she does do is Thermage, which also hurts and is also expensive, but she thinks it's better value.

It's all so overwhelming, right?

Some other dermatologists say that women our age might want to consider spending money on just three things. One: a good zinc sunscreen, worn every day like it's going out of style. Two: treti-noin (Retin-A) cream every night. (If you're doing this, you'll probably want to skip the toner, or wait a half hour after you use it to apply the tretinoin.) Three: Botox every few months.

The first two are relatively cheap. The third costs anywhere from $300 to about $1,000 per treatment based on what part of the world you live in and how fancy your doctor's office is. And Botox can freeze some facial expressions, which many women might not want. The first time I did it, I had to go off and do a horror film, and my looks of terror were definitely compromised. But I'd wanted to try it because my friend had done it and looked so great. Since then I've only done "baby Botox" between shoots, but I'm always researching new things to try.

The makeup we can wear also changes as we age. When I was shooting sixteen hours a day on *Gypsy*, my makeup artist, Kyra Panchenko, and I were waging a constant battle against redness and irritation on my skin. "It's easy to do people with young skin. You can literally slap anything on their face and they look good," she said. "But with an older woman, you have to really take the time and care. Some brushes that used to be fine are too rough on older skin."

Mary Wiles, a makeup artist to many celebrities, says the key to makeup at this age is "keeping the skin really fresh and dewy and not too much powder, not too much base."

She says, "A strong brow always looks youthful, because as we start to age our eyes get hooded and our eyebrows thin out." To combat this, she recommends lash definition via a lot of mascara and a little bit of liner on the lash line, a dark brown or black.

She uses an eyelash curler to make the eyes look more open and a nice matte tone of eye shadow without too much iridescence. "Natural makeup in the tones you have in your skin will enhance what you already have. If you have a blue-tone lip don't put on an orange lipstick. Keep your color palette cool." She also likes a cream blush rather than a powder. She says, "I feel like the market is flooded with powders, and no one really wants to use them." Powder sinks into crevices, and if you have a lot of wrinkles, it can look "like your face is cracking off." Lip liner helps with definition, and if you're pale you might consider wearing a bold lipstick.

Bobbi Brown, who's been in the field for forty years, told me, "In terms of beauty, I really just started figuring out what to do with makeup so I don't look tired, so I look prettier in my skin. As we get older, most of us get drier. Moisture is the key. I don't go anywhere without an oil stick because when I look dry and dehydrated, I probably am, so I just throw the oil on."

Essentially, an oil stick is a face oil or serum you can carry around in your purse and rub into your skin when you're feeling dried out or when you develop a dry patch. For a budget option, I like L'Oréal's Lumi Glotion.

I also know of some good makeup hacks, including eyebrow and lash tint, and an array of highlighters. I always get compliments when I use my Westman Atelier highlighter, which fully absorbs, so it doesn't rub off on your hair and make it greasy. Bobbi Brown's brand, Jones Road, has a great moisturizer that also highlights, called Miracle Balm.

Brown told me, "I don't wear traditional foundations. I wear the foundation I make because it is full of moisture and gives me a lift. I always need blush. I think as we get older, blush is our best friend, and I just go right for a bright pink color. I'll put something on top of it to give it a little sparkle, and if everything else fades away, I have that. I'm not a lipstick person. I don't love myself in lipstick. But I absolutely define my eyes. I want my brows a little stronger. I want liner. I want black mascara."

I've noticed that she also wears stylish glasses. So many women I know begin wearing bold frames in middle age, and they also start experimenting with progressive lenses. You know you're ready for progressives—lenses that incorporate multiple prescriptions for close-up, intermediate, and far distances—if you have more than one pair of glasses and have to keep switching them. If you put on reading glasses to read a menu and then put on your other glasses to read the specials on the board, or if you have trouble reading your dashboard GPS without lifting up your distance glasses while driving, it might be time to consider progressives.

Some people hate progressives, because they can take some time to acclimate to and there can be blurriness in your peripheral vision. But there's less adjustment involved if you start wearing them as soon as you begin needing them rather than later, when your prescription is stronger. And once you get used to them, they can be lifesavers, giving you seamlessly perfect vision like you had when you were younger.

I wish that society didn't force-feed us the idea that women must try to look ten years younger at all times, whereas men look more interesting and rugged and powerful as they age. I hate that messaging. I do what I can to debunk it, but in terms of doing little things here and there—or big things, for that matter—to help you feel your best, I say, Why not? No judgment ever!

One friend told me that her aging face totally preoccupies her. When she sees photos of herself, she sees only her wrinkles, so she tries to shoot herself exclusively from above. I have other friends who take great pride in their lines. I fall somewhere in between. I felt such a load lifting when I started speaking out about the aging process, but that doesn't mean that I'm immune to the hazards of self-scrutiny. Obviously when I'm on camera and expected to look my best, I work hard at it. I'm very aware of lighting and face angles. And until I'm convinced that some good face work would be better than great lighting and good angles, I'll probably keep doing my research on plastic surgery, and likely holding off. But I never say never. In fact, some days I'm quite sure I'll be putting it in the books!

Usually I'm glad I can still play a wide range of characters because my face is still expressive. In *Feud: Capote vs. The Swans*, I got to play the age range of forty to sixty-three. I am my age, and my face represents that. And what I bring to a story or a character represents that, too. I've experienced grief. I've experienced loss. I've experienced a major breakup, and I felt so much shame about having a broken family, even knowing that my ex and I are both in happy, healthier relationships and our kids love their new family members. I still feel a sense of failure sometimes.

And so that's the kind of woman I'm going to play, one who's made sacrifices and hard decisions. I'm not going to be playing someone who's falling in love for the first time. So why shouldn't I just embrace this and own it? It's fair to say I'm all over the place on this issue—sometimes for cosmetic interventions and sometimes against. I just hope society can get to a place where it can handle a woman who looks her age. I'm counting on people to adjust their tolerance rather than my having to adjust my jowls.

Things They Really Should Tell Us
About Our Midlife Skin and Hair

- Your skin looks different at fifty than it did at twenty because of slower cellular turnover. We can use retinoids or exfoliants to encourage faster turnover, but we have to balance that with proper moisturizing.

- Dry skin is common in menopause, but 25 percent of women ages forty through forty-nine are still suffering with acne.

- One recommended midlife regimen is a zinc sunscreen in the morning and Retin-A at night.

- Sleep is important for healthy skin. So is loads of water.

- A woman's hair part widens with age, and treatments, including hair-matching powders, are available to hide a visible scalp.

- It's important to see a dermatologist who understands menopause. Dryness in particular can be helped by estrogen.

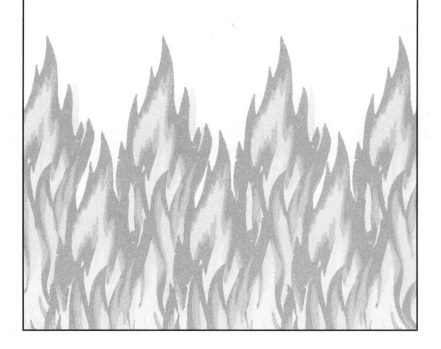

CHAPTER TEN

AWAKE AT
3:00 A.M.

"Sleep more!" everyone tells us, as if that will be the solution to all our problems. Even I have been recommending better sleep throughout these pages ad nauseam. We've probably all tried that, along with a million other things. The sleep-more-drink-more-water-exercise-more messaging can get infuriating. *I know I should!* I want to shout. But *how?*

It came to pass as I found myself entering middle age: I *could not sleep.* It felt, in fact, like I had never slept in my entire life. I couldn't remember the last time I hadn't woken up at 3:00 a.m., and maybe also at 1:00 a.m. and 5:00 a.m.—if I was able to fall asleep at all. My kids were two and four. I'd already been through a lot of sleeplessness, getting up with them when they were babies. But by that point, the kids were at least sort of sleeping. Why couldn't I?

You'd think we'd get used to it after a while, adapt to sleeplessness like people in cold climates adapt to snow. But I did not. I was and remain terrible at functioning with no sleep. Maybe I can manage one night, but then two, three in a row, and I'm a dog's breakfast, as we say in the United Kingdom.

Dr. Suzanne Gilberg-Lenz said this can be one of the most insidious parts of menopause: "I delivered babies for twenty-two years, so I know what kind of a person I am if I don't sleep. It took me a long time to be able to say to people in my life, my kids, my partner, 'Today is not the day. I'm going to be a raving maniac, and I'm only going to want carbs. So just stay away from me right now.' I would just get home from work, and I'd say, 'I don't know how to talk right now.'" The less she slept, the more she found it hard to be present for her family.

My friend Lisa told me that sleeplessness for her was the worst symptom of menopause: "My first indication that something was different was when my usual 3:00 a.m. wake-ups would last till dawn. It was like I had done a massive line of speed; I was so wired. I would then stumble through the day somehow, thinking that it was just all the grief and stress in my life, as I was caring for pre-teens and a mother with dementia.

"It wasn't till I had thoughts of divorcing my husband—whom I actually loved and still very much do—for his loud breathing and basically EVERY WORD THAT CAME OUT OF HIS MOUTH, that I realized that this may be more than just stress. I still never thought it could be hormonal, as it was never much discussed amongst my friends and I still had my period, albeit lightly.

"Luckily for me I rang my obstetrician and began to tell him what was happening. He didn't even let me finish my lack of sleep complaint before he said, 'You are coming in to see me first thing Monday morning. I am no longer an obstetrician. I am actually the head of Australia's menopause society.'

"*Bang!* All my fears around breast cancer were dispelled. He showed me data, explained the benefits of HRT for heart, bone density, and sleep health, as well as the downside of ignoring it all and being 'stoic' like our poor mothers, who, let's face it, lost not only their minds but often their marriages and friendships, too. I, luckily, was never prone to depression, but my darling mum was, and menopause tipped her over the edge. I thank God I called my doctor that day."

Doctors will usually work with you to come up with a combination of sleep hygiene, HRT, sleep aids, and other treatments until a solution is found. Lisa's doctor put her on estrogen gel and progesterone tablets. And for her that made all the difference: "Overnight my life turned around—sleep came back, my husband suddenly became a quiet breather, and my friends didn't annoy me." Progesterone, known as the "relaxing hormone," taken before bed can purportedly have a sedative effect.

Hormone therapy hasn't completely solved my sleep problems, though I believe progesterone really has helped me. Maybe there's just no going back to the kind of sleep we had when we were young. How is it possible that at one time I could fall asleep on anyone's couch, sleep the whole night, and wake up fully clothed and perfectly well rested but now the conditions need to be perfect, and even then I'm up multiple times?

Like a lot of people, I've found tracking my sleep has helped me prioritize it, the same way using a step counter tends to get us to walk more. To track my sleep, I've been using a device called the Oura Ring (which retails for about three hundred dollars; the Fitbit is more affordable). Worn on your finger, it tracks your biometrics and tells you how much sleep you get, and what kind of quality it is. I found it became a journal of sorts, by which I was able to notice patterns and see where change might be needed. (All forms of journaling can prove helpful in this way, whether it's keeping track of diet, mood, or symptoms.)

Sleep doctors I've spoken with say sleep trackers might over-promise when they tell you exactly what amount of time you spend in each sleep stage, but I've become addicted to seeing my report every morning. According to my ring, I get six to seven and a half hours of sleep a night, and my deep sleep is nearly always under an hour and never more than one hour and fifteen minutes. The rest is a combo of REM and light sleep, with lots of waking up in between.

I called Dr. Suzie Bertisch, clinical director of Behavioral Sleep Medicine at Brigham and Women's Hospital and assistant professor of medicine at Harvard Medical School, to see what I might be able to do to sleep better. Her clinical expertise is insomnia, though she treats all sleep disorders.

"My interest in insomnia during menopause really grew when I started to do research studies with Dr. Hadine Joffe," she told me. "She's one of the prominent scientists in sleep in menopause. In the physiology study we were doing, I had the role of interviewing women with what we call 'hot-flash-associated insomnia' or an insomnia disorder that started or worsened during the menopause transition. This was an intensive physiology study of about forty women, but all were in some stage of menopause and twenty-five had menopause-related insomnia. When I spoke with the women with insomnia, a condition I was treating regularly in my clinical practice, I was struck by the stories I heard about why they had not yet received treatment. Many women recalled, they were told by their doctors that this was just the natural phase of life, and there's nothing more you can do about it. Shrug your shoulders, grin and bear it. That's what really opened my eyes. I realized the gap between what we know about treating insomnia with the information these women were receiving. We have treatment to help people sleep better!"

She said menopause-related sleep issues can feel challenging to treat because, while part is likely physical and can be treated through hormones or other pharmacologic treatments for hot flashes, there are plenty of other issues that fall outside the medical realm that impact sleep, like childcare demands or caring for older parents, what Dr. Bertisch calls "a big mesh of biological, social, and environmental demands that unfortunately all happen at once." Causes for poor sleep, like causes for low libido, could be any combination of physical, emotional, mental, and situational. "However, despite these constraints, we do have evidence-based tools to help women sleep better," she said.

"When we see a woman with menopause or perimenopause in our clinic, when we think about sleep disruption, we need to do a full evaluation," Dr. Bertisch told me. "When women hit menopause, their risk of sleep apnea goes up. Restless legs syndrome, too, as well as other conditions that impact sleep, such as mood disorders. These are all things that can cause disruptive sleep or insomnia symptoms."

She recommends various behavioral and practical strategies to reset the brain and get it ready for sleep but warns that many of the practical strategies you read about on the internet, which are often referred to as "sleep hygiene," might be necessary to improve sleep but have been shown to be ineffective as stand-alone treatment of patients with insomnia disorder. So while these recommendations, such as avoiding caffeine late in the day and lowering the temperature of the room to around 65 degrees Fahrenheit (when possible) can be tried, this is only a starting point to help promote sleep in women with sleep problems during the menopause transition. For patients with persistent problems, there is evidence supporting the use of cognitive behavioral therapy (or CBT-I) among women with insomnia, including sleep problems associated with hot flashes. CBT-I is often misrepresented as talk therapy, but it targets both behavioral change and cognitive therapy focused specifically on sleep. This incorporates a combination of strategies, including changing behaviors to reduce time awake in bed, establishing regular sleep routines, reducing thoughts that interfere with sleep, and giving relaxation techniques a try. For instance, in CBT-I, patients learn to pay attention and manipulate their "homeostatic sleep drive," or "sleep hunger," meaning the longer we're awake, the hungrier we are for sleep. "It is what we feel if we stay up way past our usual bedtime; we'll feel sleepy and it's usually easier to fall asleep." Yes, she means stay up later. She also tells patients with insomnia that once you're in bed, if you're having trouble sleeping, get out of bed and wait until you feel sleepy again so you don't train your brain to associate the bed with not sleeping.

Then of course there are always drugs.

I feel like almost everybody I know is taking some kind of sleep aid. The most common class is the benzodiazepines, like the anti-anxiety drug Klonopin (clonazepam). It has a sedative effect, and even though it can cause dependence or tolerance over time, and there might be an increased risk of cognitive decline or falls, I don't see that stopping many people I know. Another category is drugs that work on the same receptor as benzodiazepines like Ambien (zolpidem), which have a shorter half-life but carry an FDA black box warning. Sometimes, especially in combination with alcohol (which also works on the same receptor), they can cause people to act very strangely.

I have experienced this firsthand. When I flew to Milan for a fashion show, I knew I had to have a full night of sleep, and the time difference was making me nervous. So I took an Ambien my first night at the hotel to ensure I'd get eight hours of sleep in order to look half-decent for the event. The next day, I woke to find that I had eaten the entire contents of the minibar. I had no memory of eating anything, but there was plenty of evidence that I had. Wrappers were everywhere. And looking at my phone, I found multiple photos of me eating everything. Apparently, Ambien-me thought what I was doing was hilarious. Needless to say, that was the last time I took Ambien. I decided that one was *not* for me.

Finally, there are "sedating antidepressants," like trazodone. Then, of course, some people swear by magnesium, melatonin, or cannabinoids. I try to avoid taking sleeping pills as much as I can, but in an emergency, I will take them short-term. I would first try melatonin, Advil PM, or Benadryl. And if I need something stronger, I'd make a thirty-day prescription last a full two years. Using sleep aids can be a slippery slope.

Dr. Bertisch said, "Melatonin is actually useful for jet lag. When you're traveling east, you could take it at your desired bedtime in the new location."

One caveat: melatonin falls into the category of dietary supplements, which are unregulated in the United States, so pill to pill, the dose varies. But most of the doctors I spoke with agree that of all the supplements out there, melatonin is probably one of the safer ones.

"Some of these medications, like the benzodiazepines, Ambien, and Lunesta (eszopiclone), have been tested in women with menopause and can improve sleep," Dr. Bertisch told me. "Suvorexant, which is a newer class of medication, has modest impacts on sleep in women with hot-flash-associated insomnia."

Of course, as with any medication, there are trade-offs. Sleeping pills may cause cognitive decline or dependence. But it's good to bear in mind that getting very little sleep is its own risk factor! As with HRT, you might try many things before finding the best one for you. "The problem is a lot of physicians aren't taught about menopause or sleep, and they're supposed to provide answers," said Dr. Bertisch. "How you choose medications really depends on the patient. Are there other medical issues? What are the patient's preferences? Do they only want to be on medications, do they not want medications? Is there a combination of treatments? It can be confusing to know what to suggest."

And yet, there are a few remedies with no risk that sleep doctors suggest pretty universally:

1. Establish a Routine

"Some people need more sleep than others, but bodies like natural rhythms and sleep patterns," said Dr. Bertisch. "So, wake up and go to bed at the same times each day. When we open our eyes in the morning and the natural light hits us, that's what sets our rhythm for the next twenty-four-ish hours."

2. Wind Down

Start the sleep process hours before getting into bed. Many experts suggest putting more than an hour or two between bedtime and your last meal, alcoholic drink, or exposure to screens. So many people look at their phones before bed, but all sleep doctors seem to think that's a bad idea.

Dr. Bertisch told me that if you eat a big meal late in the day and you're prone to heartburn, you're probably not going to sleep as well just because of the discomfort or gas.

3. Exercise

We all know this, but it's scientifically proven: If you get more exercise during the day, it's likely you'll have better sleep quality at night.

4. Don't Drink

I sometimes like wine with dinner, so I don't love hearing this, but it's hard to argue with the research. Alcohol can help us fall asleep, but then it causes us to wake up more during the night. While alcohol is still in your system, it has a calming effect, so you'll sleep hard. But as it leaves your body, you have what's called "rebound arousal." That means you might wake up or have nightmares.

I know that drinking will interfere with my sleep and even my memory, which is why I don't drink when I'm filming. But when I'm in between jobs, or on a weekend, sometimes I just say, "I'm going to have that extra glass of wine with my friends," because it feels nice in the moment.

Dr. Mary Claire Haver confirms what I've found to be true in my own life: "If you drink alcohol, you may be choosing not to sleep. That is me and the majority of my patients. Sleep is already disrupted from menopause. Even with HRT, it's never going to be the same."

Certainly, I've found that if I have more than one glass of wine, especially later in the evening, I am making a conscious decision that I'm going to sacrifice my sleep. I'm going to be up at three.

"If you're not sleeping, your memory's going to take a hit as well," says Dr. Haver. "And for menopausal symptoms that stem from the brain, like brain fog and anxiety, alcohol seems to exacerbate the severity of these. Furthermore, alcohol can make hot flashes worse, and hot flashes and temperature regulation are the most likely symptoms to disrupt a woman's sleep. But even if a woman doesn't have hot flashes, her sleep can be disrupted. The anxiety, the racing thoughts, and the mental health symptoms at night can lead to difficulty falling asleep. Also, a woman wakes up in the middle of the night courtesy of her bladder. If you have incontinence or an overactive bladder and it's not treated, you will have to get up and pee and then may struggle to fall back asleep."

Also, alcohol makes sleep apnea worse and can lead to more snoring. If sleep is a problem, it's worth thinking about taking a break from drinking, or at least being sure to stop a couple of hours before bed.

The upshot: if you can't sleep, you're far from alone and you might have to prioritize figuring out what your sleep issues are and finding the right treatment or making lifestyle adjustments. I know it's not easy, especially when you're irritable from the sleep deprivation itself! But doctors who know about menopause should work with you to find a solution.

Things They Really Should Tell Us About Better Sleep

- You can use an Oura Ring, Fitbit, or smart watch to keep track of your sleep.
- There are many sleep-aid drugs, each with their own pros and cons. Melatonin is recommended for jet lag.
- Sleep hygiene includes getting off screens, eating your last meal of the day, and stopping alcohol consumption at least a couple of hours before going to bed.
- Exercise will help you sleep better at night.
- Get on a routine that makes sense for you.
- Let in natural light to help your body know when to wake up.

CHAPTER ELEVEN

CLOSET
CONFIDENTIAL

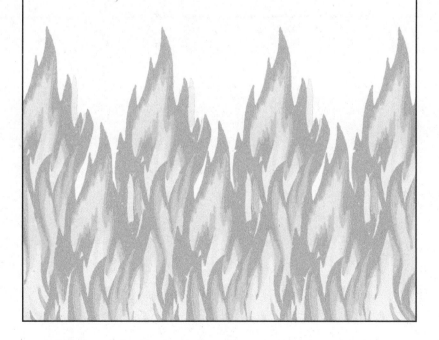

"**M**y decision to stop coloring my hair was disturbing to my patients," said Dr. Suzanne Gilberg-Lenz. "I'm not kidding. They said, 'Are you *okay*?' Or 'You know, you could do highlights.' I said, 'I'm fifty-three. I'm aware that it's possible not to have gray hair. I decided to do this. I realize to you it might look weird.' Some of my patients were truly disturbed, I think because, if we were the same age, seeing me like that made them feel old."

And yet, many women, with their regular schedules at the salon disrupted by Covid, went gray during lockdown and ended up loving it. Dyeing your hair takes a whole lot of time and money, and once you realize it's not necessary, it becomes harder to go back. I've reduced coloring my hair to twice a year. Luckily, my grays don't show so easily with blond hair.

I see a lot of women my age rethinking how they present themselves to the world, in terms of their hair or their makeup or their clothing.

"The only way to maintain a sense of personal style as we age is to accept that we are aging and our bodies are changing," the stylist Stacy London told me. "Style is not static. It must evolve as we do or we get stuck in the idea that who we were is the *only* version of ourselves. Personal style is personal if it is about you as you are, today. That means that things must and will change!"

For example, you may need a new color palette to better match changes to your hair or skin.

"It's not simply your body that's changing; your taste and perception will change, too," Stacy said. "A style that was once a cornerstone of your look may no longer feel comfortable or even appealing to you. This is not about grieving your youth. It's about being your age and the possibility surrounding a new style. Try approaching that process with wonder and curiosity rather than grief.

Everything about personal style should be geared toward your happiness and comfort at any age."

For me, if I wear a bikini it's not a string bikini. I'll make sure it's high-waisted, covering my belly button. And for a time I hid my thighs after a trainer I'd worked with described them in his book as "fleshy." It got in my head! (I'm glad I don't have to see my own elbows, so I'll wear whatever sleeves I want and if you need to look away, that's your problem!)

There are no universal rules. We should wear whatever we want, especially in middle age. I know one woman who felt she had to stop wearing animal prints when she got older and another who decided she needed to spice things up and *started* wearing animal prints. One woman in her fifties told me, "I don't believe that whole thing where you have to dress your age and cut your hair and all of that. I mean, at this point who exactly am I dressing for?"

My stylist, Jeanann Williams, says older women often want to stop baring their stomachs around this age, but she also says that what we love about our bodies should become our focus, even if it's our midriff: "If you've got great gams or a killer rack, play them up as long as they hold up, I say!"

Friends of mine complain about their changing bodies. "Social media seems to recognize I'm desperate and keeps pushing ads for wall Pilates to help get rid of 'menopause belly,'" one grumbled to me the other day.

Fashion-advice columns often feature women in menopause grappling with "belly bulge" or "widening," as well as with a tendency to overheat. *New York Times* critic Vanessa Friedman wrote in her column about dressing for middle age that in addition to layering, it makes sense to wear separates and breathable fabrics "like cotton, linen, and bamboo." (My mum has been wearing fabulous caftans in textured linen or fantastic prints for years; they always cheer me up. Playing Babe Paley, I got to swan about in some silky ones. I am definitely ready for my muumuu era.)

Friedman's tips include: "A crew neck sweater over a shirt with a structured blazer and scarf with jeans (high- or low-waist, depending on your comfort zone) looks polished, and pieces can be added or discarded at will. If you no longer love your upper arms, slip a long-sleeved, leotard-like top or bodysuit beneath your sleeveless tops. Well-tailored jackets cover any stomach sensitivities you may have. Why do you think men have been wearing them for so long?"

Friedman notes, too, that it's helpful to find a reasonably priced tailor who can adjust your clothes, and to ignore sizes and just try on a lot of stuff. Sizes vary so widely across brands—you might be an 8 in one clothing brand and a 12 in another—that they're borderline meaningless.

Finally, she says that the eye is drawn to the most brightly colored, sparkly things, so to draw attention away from your middle, if that's what you're feeling shy about, you can try a beaded top or colorful scarf or attention-getting jewelry.

At least the pressure to wear high heels seems to be off. I think the pandemic got a lot of us out of heels, and then it was harder to go back. There are plenty of formal flats. I love the trend of women at formal events wearing suits with fashionable sneakers.

The key word I heard again and again talking to menopausal women about fashion was "liberation."

"I think what's changed about my approach to fashion is that I'm less interested in trends, and I'm less interested in buying a lot," Stacy London told me. "I buy what suits me, not what the runways look like. I buy fewer pieces of higher quality that I know I can integrate in my wardrobe for several seasons, not simply one. I make sure that if I am buying a single piece, it already goes with at least two to three other items in my closet.

"If I'm not sure, I prefer to buy in outfits rather than pieces so that I always know I have something that works immediately rather than having to try and style it later. I can always mix and match pieces at home, of course. But just think of that one piece you bought on its own and never figured out what to wear it with (maybe you have more than one!). Don't leave strays to sit there. Find pieces that help you make complete outfits with what you already own. You'll spend less time worrying about what to wear!

"Lastly, everything I buy has to meet at least one of two criteria, hopefully both. It has to have use value and bring me joy. If it doesn't meet either of those criteria, I leave it behind."

Stacy also delivered these good tidings: "Believe it or not, I think the fashion industry is starting to pay attention to women in midlife and beyond. Just like the plus-size industry, we have to rid ourselves of a lot of cultural biases around ageism and prove there is a market for the clothes. There are *a lot* of women with buying power who don't want to look like their daughters and who still want to feel relevant, chic, and sexy as hell. Even as we age, even as our bodies change, feeling your best isn't a privilege, it's a right. More and more companies (some old and some new!) are paying attention, and that is going to change the game."

The great liberation for me has been realizing that when it comes to how we look, as the saying goes, the people "who mind don't matter, and those who matter don't mind."

I've also banished the phrase "age appropriate" from my lexicon. Appropriate for what? Says who? Look at Vivienne Westwood! She was innovating with materials and silhouettes right up until the end, and we loved her for it. Was she doing something wrong because she was focused on the joy of clothing? Absolutely not! After all, shouldn't clothes be fun?

Things They Really Should Tell Us About Fashion as We Age

- Gray hair can be totally fashionable!

- There are no "problem areas." Your body is your body. Play up what you love about it! Artfully hide whatever you don't.

- There are no fixed rules for how you should dress at any given age. Clothes should be about joy and personal expression, not trying to be "age appropriate."

- Sizes vary widely across brands. Finding an affordable tailor can be a huge asset.

Stacy London's Shopping List

- Denim in different silhouettes: wide-leg jeans, bootcut, flare, skinny, low-rise, high-rise. They all work with something.

- Leather (or vegan leather) pants or leggings. (A word about vegan leather: it is not all good quality. If you don't want to wear leather, make sure what you are buying won't melt on a heated car seat.)

- Crew necks that fit well.

- An oversize turtleneck, cardigan, and V-neck sweater (especially in cashmere or Cashfeel).

- A white silk or cotton button-down.

- A well-fitted suit, ideally a three-piece one with a vest or skirt option for versatility.

- A good coat (I love a statement one).

CHAPTER TWELVE

MENOBOSS

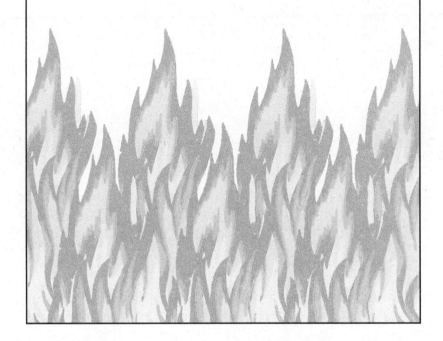

I've always had a strong sense of resilience and have been pretty good about not letting fear take hold of me. My friends and I often remark that good things happen when we take chances on ourselves. Sometimes I look back on choices I made early on in my career and think, *Wow, that was bold.* Still, not everything made sense as it was happening. Every woman I know has a winding road from where she started out to where she ended up. This is mine:

After giving up on early teen dreams of acting, I started my fashion career at nineteen, working with my costume-designer mother as a wardrobe assistant for film and TV. Then I got a styling job at a department store called Grace Bros., trying to make boring bits of apparel look good. That meant asking, *What was the concept? Where would you shoot it? Who would you hire to shoot it? Who were the models, the photographer?*

That job also led to offers to work at a magazine called *Follow Me,* which was in the realm of *Vogue* and *Harper's Bazaar.* I became the fashion editor's assistant. About a year into that, there was talk of me becoming fashion editor of a junior magazine called *Hero.*

I was working there when a friend of mine called me up and said, "Oh, will you do this acting workshop this weekend? Just do it as a favor?" I said, "No. I'm not acting anymore. I quit." Then he pleaded: "We are really short on women. The ratio's off, and it's just a weekend! Please!"

My boyfriend was away at the time. Eventually, I thought, *Okay, yeah, fine. I'll just do it.* And by the end of the weekend, both the teacher and all the other fellow actors had said, "You're living a lie. This is your dream, it's so obvious. You're so good at it. You've got to get back in the game."

This was a meaningful weekend. I did think, *Maybe they're right? It sure was fun.* Then on Monday morning, I went to my boss and said, "I'm leaving because I want to be an actor." And he said, "Ha. You can still be an actor on the weekends. Don't quit, though. Don't be ridiculous. You're at the beginning of your career, you've got a fantastic job, a great salary. You're on the road somewhere. Don't throw it all away."

"No, I'm so sorry," I said. "I'm serious. I'll stay for another month. I'll train someone, but this is what I want to do." He looked at me like I was insane. And then a handful of weeks later, I went to a casting for the movie *Flirting* and got the job. So that was that. And I started working as an actor. But I wonder where I'd be now if I hadn't said yes to that friend. The takeaway here for me is that, as they say, it's better to be at the bottom of a ladder you want to climb than halfway up one you don't.

Relocating to America was also a very bold move. I had $2,000 to my name and one phone number, belonging to a friend of my mother's. And I was friendly but not yet besties with Nicole Kidman. We'd worked together on *Flirting,* and we knew each other peripherally from back home in Australia. We became much better acquainted once I moved here. And over time I made more friends and built a community.

The point is: I was brave back then. So I can be brave now when it comes to taking risks in life. We took chances when we were younger, and didn't we know so much less back then? Midlife is a good time to bet on ourselves again.

Lately I see women all around me looking back on their careers and asking questions about what it all means and what's next.

When I've spoken to women about what it's like to be working as a menopausal woman, I've heard responses all over the map. Some are thriving. They've been in the business long enough to know their value and their power while still being young enough to have the energy to keep charging ahead.

"In midlife, men buy motorcycles or fast cars and women get PhDs," my friend Mariella Frostrup told me when I called her for her take. "A lot of men seem to slightly slow down at this age, and they're looking toward retirement and taking up golf. And women just seem to become so much more driven and ambitious and focused as our oxytocin goes down, and we lose that love for toddlers, and our children leave home. And that's an opportunity. As men slow down and head to the golf course, here we are ready to take over!"

I have several friends who were so liberated by the empty nest. They suddenly had way more energy to focus on their work and hit their prime career years when their kids were in college or later. It's a real phenomenon, and we should talk about it more, rather than just focusing on how much we miss our kids when they leave home (even if that's true, too!).

My friend Sophie recently told me, "The mothers among us will never stop worrying about or caring for our kids, but the child-rearing years of 'mother guilt' should be finally set aside. The best middle-aged mother now must surely be the one who attempts to let go—trusts in her children, after the primary job has been done. She has earned the confidence to advise on what is yet to be navigated, and hopefully with a sense of humor."

She sent me this Kahlil Gibran quote:

Your children are not your children
They are the sons and daughters of life's longing for itself
They come through you but not from you
And though they are with you yet they belong not to you

In this phase of life, Mariella Frostrup has spent the past ten years campaigning for better recognition, support, and education for menopause, having made a BBC documentary, cowritten a book called *Cracking the Menopause,* and chaired the advocacy group Menopause Mandate. Advocacy work like Mariella's is part of what's pushing forward the dialogue about every aspect of this transition, especially related to the workplace. I've known her for twenty years, and we've become incredibly close. We're comrades in our commitment to create change for women.

So many women I know had flourishing careers until they

became mothers and wound up struggling to keep everything balanced.

"That whole joke about having it all actually wears a bit thin," Mariella told me, "when you look at the economic impact of motherhood on women. Within twelve years of having your first child, you're likely to be earning 33 percent less than a male contemporary who was doing the same thing at the point you had the child. By the time you get to your pension at the end of your working life, it's going to be somewhere between 15 and 40 percent less again than that of a male contemporary."

Of course, a lot of women step out of the workplace for caregiving, for children, or for aging parents. That can put us in a terrible bind when we return to work, especially if we're having overwhelming menopause symptoms. Surrounded by younger people coming up behind us, we can struggle with confidence.

"If you decide to take three years off from paid work to do something in the domestic sphere, it is going to have an impact on your skill set," Mariella said. "It is going to have an impact on what you have to offer. Things change very quickly. But I do think for women reentering the workforce, particularly in middle age, there is an increasing understanding that they bring skills they wouldn't have had earlier.

"And if you compare what a twenty-five-year-old or even a thirty-year-old at work has to offer in terms of experience and the way they conduct themselves in the professional world, I think there is a growing realization that you need yin and yang. You need older people who can hand down experience, and you need young people who are eager to learn and feed off that experience. Only by endlessly going on about these issues will society shift. And it's not going to happen overnight, and it's not going to happen without women."

Working with people whose values you share makes everything so much easier. I believe that film is ultimately a director's medium, so I've always done my best to find directors I trust and to put myself in their capable hands. Of course, it's a collaborative experience, but the director is the main storyteller. As an actor, you have to give yourself over to their point of view as much as possible. You don't always have that luxury when the A-list directors stop calling—which has been my experience for years at a time. Maybe that's because I've had a few bombs along the way. More than a handful!

The fact is, it's rare and extremely difficult to make a film or TV show that works on all levels. Mostly they fail. And when you've been working in the industry as long as I have, you know it's all ups and downs. You are hot, and then you are not. That is the cycle. We're mostly like cicadas who spend most years underground and then on occasion get to come out and play. There's no point in getting bitter or twisted about it. You just have to keep going. So, I tend to look for a strong director and great female characters. Who are they? What are they doing? What emotional transformations are they going through? What can they teach me? How will they help me grow?

When I was starting out as an actor, I was warned to hold off on playing a mother, and certainly not to play one too often, because doing so would jeopardize my chances of playing an ingenue again. But I didn't have any qualms about that. My approach was "I want to work. I want to tell stories. I love that there are opportunities available."

Then, in 2001, came the David Lynch movie *Mulholland Drive*, which I think of as my launching pad. I always speak about my acting career in two parts, before that movie and after. Well, it wasn't much of a career before. I was more a journeyman actor, and I was okay with that. I thought that if I could keep going, just on one job a year, and pay my rent, I'd be happy. And I would have been.

But *Mulholland Drive* was when things changed for me. I'd never seen myself as a femme fatale kind of woman. But David Lynch saw me as his own version of that—or maybe more in the line of girl-next-door-on-the-verge-of-a-nervous-breakdown-who-had-a-sexual-awakening. I went from there to *The Ring*, where I was a mother of a ten-year-old; and then, in my late forties, I wound up on the TV show *Gypsy*. That's when I met Billy and played that sexually curious therapist. You just never know where you will wind up when you keep following your instincts and taking chances. Speaking up about my experience with menopause was another big career risk. But I feel like I got ahead of it. Naming what someone is thinking before they say it has let me own my vulnerability as my power. And I've been given terrific roles since I became vocal on this subject, including on *Feud: Capote vs. The Swans* and in *The Friend* and *All's Fair*.

Of course I've often played older, as women often do. In the Divergent series, I played the mother of Theo James. While we were shooting, he had a birthday. I didn't realize how close we were in age until he had a cake on set with thirty candles. Gulp. If I have my math right, I was only about sixteen years older than he was. He later told an interviewer, "It was interesting because she's playing my mum, but she's a bit of a babe. I had to get past that." (And, yes, when I read that interview, I blushed scarlet.) So that's another reason to avoid casting women to play much older than they are: so you don't get "interesting" mother-son chemistry. (But thank you for the compliment, Theo!)

I know my career story is about a strange job not a lot of people have, but I feel like there are versions of these twists and turns in every industry. And I believe that whatever work we do, the same principles apply—trust your instincts and take chances.

Approximately 75 percent of women ages forty-five to fifty-five are working. That's a lot of women who are dealing with their aging bodies and complex middle-aged lives in the arena of the workplace. How can we support ourselves, take the chances we need to take, and show the world what we are capable of? It's in our interest and our employers' interests for our workplaces to be menopause friendly, and, fortunately, flexible scheduling, remote work, and shared parental leave are becoming more common. While the UK was leading the way for a long time, it feels like the United States is finally catching up.

One of the most memorable stories I've heard about being in the workplace as a menopausal woman comes from Tamsen Fadal. She'd been doing local news for thirty years. On a Friday night, about three minutes before the end of a commercial break, her heart started racing. She'd had some brain fog, but she'd chalked it up to stress. This time, though, it was that plus a blind panic. She thought she might throw up. She said to the men in the studio, "If I fall over, someone catch me."

"The sports anchor took one look at me and said, 'I think you should get off the set.' I'd never left a live set in thirty years of working in television. He helped me off. I went to the bathroom. I lay on the floor and shut my whole body down." Her co-anchor finished the show alone.

She'd been living off almost no sleep for a long time, and it had never been a problem. But something had shifted. And from that night in the studio on, she was plagued by self-doubt: *When is it going to happen again?* That was always the fear. "So, that's when I started a deep dive on my health. I made an appointment with my doctor. I did all sorts of tests, and then the doctor sent me a little note on my patient portal that said, 'In menopause. Any questions?' That was it."

Of course, she did have questions, but they went unanswered for a long time. The doctor told her, "There's probably some solutions, but most women just get through it. It'll be a few years."

Just suffer for a few years. Risk freezing up live on air.

Finally, she found a new doctor who said, "Your hot flashes are indications of something. This brain fog is indication of something. You need to handle these things, not just for your comfort, not just so you don't suffer, but for your long-term health."

After going on hormone therapy, she felt more like herself, and she no longer feared having an episode at work. But that experience had started her on a journey, and now she realized that she was at a significant crossroads; there was more she wanted to do in her life.

I find Tamsen so inspiring. Fear of failure is a toxic thing to carry, and yet that is what many women do. But Tamsen didn't let her fear get in the way of trying new things. She's since left her job of fifteen years and is writing books and producing documentaries, as well as connecting with other women on the subject of menopause. And she's doing it all on her own terms.

Bobbi Brown, who started a new company in her sixties, told me, "I think anything is possible. I guess I'm not afraid, because if something doesn't work, I don't look at it as a failure. I say, *Okay, that didn't work. Let me try something else.* And I also realized that if something doesn't work, instead of being frustrated, you can just take a step back and say, 'Okay, what should I have done differently?'"

According to the social psychologist Dr. Carol Tavris, the way to navigate work during this phase of life is "First of all, get rid of the list of obligations, or what the rational emotive therapist Albert Ellis called 'musturbation.' *I must do this, and I must do that. I must do this other thing.*"

The pressure on women to be all things to all people can be overwhelming, and menopause can add an extra layer of stress. Women who took time out of the workplace to raise their kids may feel like it's a cruel joke that right when they're raring to get back to work, they're going through menopause, having to deal with symptoms exactly when they need to rally their most confident selves.

Whatever it takes for us to get our confidence up, I say! By this point in our lives, we've failed many times before. So we know how to recover, even if it's hard to do. It can be helpful to recall the ways we've bounced back in the past.

I feel more open to risk now than I ever have. For example, writing this book feels so exposing! I hate public speaking, and now here I am signing up for a book tour. (Fortunately, I've found that a little beta blocker can help.)

Whenever I experience imposter syndrome—and I still do, not just when I'm certain I'm out of my depth in different fields but even in my chosen field, in spite of how long I've been doing this work—I remember a time when I almost let it get the better of me.

I'd hit a point in my career as an actor where I was not getting jobs for a long period of time. I'd done a handful of projects and had what I thought was a great show reel. And yet I wasn't booking anything. Finally, I went to see my agent and I said, "Why am I not getting any work?"

"Do you really want to know?" she asked me. "You want the honest answer?"

I said yes.

"You're too intense. You make people feel uncomfortable with your nervousness. They pick up on that energy, and you then become not funny, not sexy, not dynamic. You want it too badly. It's coming across as desperate."

No shit, Sherlock! I am *desperate!*

I went home to my apartment, where I was two months late on my rent. My mum was staying with me at the time.

Recounting my day, I fell to pieces in her arms.

"That's not true," my mother said. "Whatever it is you are putting forward, you are not those things they're seeing. You're enough as you. Of course you're nervous—you've had five years of rejection in a row! And you're trying to reshape yourself into what you think they want. You just have to remember who you are, and eventually that will be the right version of a person that they're looking for."

That was a pivotal moment. I had to stop diluting and reshaping myself into what I imagined they wanted.

I think of that pep talk when I feel insecure. I remind myself of what I've done and who I am and why I'm in the room. I remember that it's important to challenge myself to do things that I think will be of benefit in some way to other people, even if those things fill me with anxiety. And I've found that when I act in ways that are consistent with my values, I never regret having taken the leap.

Owning your vulnerabilities always leads to a more powerful outcome. Our lived experience is meaningful and has great value for workplaces. Many of the leading midlife experts say that it's key at this point in life to find what it is we love to do and to cultivate it, and then share it. So I remind myself, and my friends when they struggle, of what my mum said: *You are enough. There's only one you.*

It took me a long time to trust in all that, but now I do—even if I need a little reminder now and again.

Things They Really Should Tell Us About Work in Midlife

- Three-quarters of menopausal women are in the workplace! This is leading many workplaces to become more menopause friendly.

- Some of the positive changes coming to workplaces include flexible scheduling, remote work, and shared parental leave.

- We should cease "musturbation." Life's too short to worry about other people's priorities.

- This is a good time of life to take risks and bet on our own abilities. Find a mantra that gives you confidence.

CHAPTER THIRTEEN

RETHINKING NUTRITION

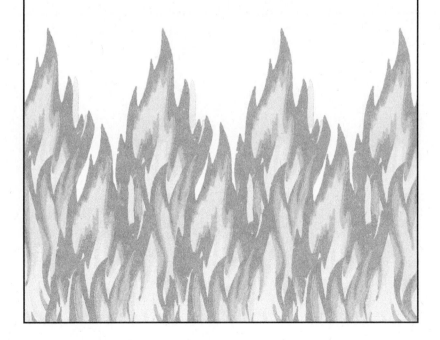

When I was about eighteen, I started modeling in Tokyo. I'd been there for about three months when the work started drying up. I went to see my agent and said, "I don't know why I'm not getting any work anymore."

"Well, you've gained too much weight," she said.

"What do you mean?" I said. I'd never been all that aware of my size up until that point, other than being annoyingly flat-chested. It was the era where we were wearing tights and big, baggy T-shirts, so it wasn't like I couldn't get my jeans closed. I had no awareness that my body had changed. It was the first time I'd been away from home. I was eating lots of pizza and junk food.

Basically, my agent said, "I think it's time for you to go."

When my mum's best friend first saw me, she said, "What? Is that you, Naomi?"

She didn't recognize me. I got on the scales and realized I'd gained more than twenty pounds in three months.

In the household in Tokyo where I was staying I was known as Yo-Yo, because the kids in the family couldn't say "Naomi." Now that I was yo-yoing between weights, that nickname took on a new resonance. After that, I felt sensitive about my weight and became a bit obsessed with fad diets through my early twenties. When I got into acting, I was afraid I'd lose jobs again the same way. I've stayed relatively slim ever since by eating healthily and working out a few times a week. I'll confess it was a challenge at times not to become obsessed with dieting. I even had to sort myself out with therapy at one point. Now that I have a healthier relationship to food, I guard it carefully.

Whenever I've tried a hard-core diet with lots of rules, I've found the restrictions bring out my rebellious streak and I'm setting myself up for failure. I might do a three-day cleanse every now and again. But I have to be able to eat salads and soups at the very

least. It's best for me to just stay in the moderate zone on everything. I won't deny myself treats like potato chips, for example, and
during Easter they basically have to back up a truck of those candy
Easter eggs to my house since I eat so many of them.

When it comes to food, I'm always wary of telling people, "This
is what works!" because everyone is different, so I'm not going to
tell you what to eat or when to eat it, but I can say what works for
me. I really try to be careful without being too strict. And recently
I've been asking doctors what they tell their patients about eating
well during menopause. At this stage of life it doesn't usually feel
the same to eat the way we did when we were teenagers!

One of these doctors is my friend Dr. Mary Claire Haver. She
is a board-certified ob-gyn in Texas, a certified culinary medicine
specialist. Her earlier book, *The Galveston Diet,* is about focusing
on becoming stronger and healthier, not necessarily thinner. She
tells women that to help manage the symptoms associated with
fluctuating estrogen levels, we should eat more broccoli, avocados,
leafy greens, fish, flax seeds, and pumpkin seeds.

She also says that we should consider overall nutrition, not just
count calories. A lot of us need more protein than we're getting.
"Right now, the FDA recommends that women need about 0.8
grams of protein per kilogram of body mass. But the newest data
from the Women's Health Initiative found that menopausal women
who eat double that amount, about 1.6 grams of protein per kilogram of body mass, had much lower fragility scores than women
who ate the recommended amount."

So many dieting women I know see "carbs" and panic, but carbs
aren't just about pasta and bread, which often contain empty calories. There are many healthy foods that contain carbs but also have
a lot of fiber, antioxidants, and vitamins, like quinoa, oats, blueberries, apples, and sweet potatoes.

Weight gain in menopause is real, and there are tons of factors
that make it so. For one thing, in menopause we tend to gain visceral fat—that's fat around the middle of our bodies—because of a
complicated interplay of hormones. Weight gain may also be con-

nected to inflammation in the body, which is why we hear so much about "anti-inflammatory diets" like the Mediterranean diet. The idea is that our bodies become inflamed in reaction to injury, but when inflammation becomes chronic, it can cause weight gain. Processed foods are thought to increase inflammation.

"Subcutaneous fat is the fat under our skin. It gives us our breasts and curves and cellulite," Dr. Haver told me. "We might not like it cosmetically, but it really isn't that dangerous. Visceral fat is the fat that is in our intrabdominal cavity and wraps around our internal organs. Through the menopause transition, we see a big shift in where we store our fat. Our visceral fat is around 8 percent on average in the premenopausal period. And then through the menopausal transition to postmenopause, it goes up to 23 percent. So, we have a three times expansion of our visceral fat cavity. Visceral fat is biologically active and inflammatory. Elevated amounts lead to increased risks of hypertension, diabetes, and stroke. I love to educate my patients and followers about strategies aimed at decreasing visceral fat. Usually, these solutions tend to be approaches most of us never considered in our nutritional strategies to stay healthy. For example, women have an average fiber intake of about 10 grams per day. However, women who enjoy 25 to 32 grams of fiber in their diets per day have lower visceral fat, lower diabetes risk, and a healthier gut microbiome.

"The keto movement tended to throw out the carbohydrate baby with the bathwater. A lot of people were avoiding all carbohydrates even though things like fruits and vegetables, legumes, nuts and seeds are not only packed with fiber, but also minerals, vitamins, and nutrients. However, women who limit *added* sugars (from cooking, processing, and alcohol) to 25 grams per day have lower visceral fat levels than women who don't."

It feels like everyone is talking about the benefits of probiotics (the good kind of bacteria) these days. I know a lot of people who take a daily probiotic, or who swear by a daily kombucha. Probiotics in whatever form are useful for keeping the right balance of good bacteria in the gut.

"In the United States most people, if they get probiotics from food, it's going to be from yogurt. However, most commercially available yogurt has a tremendous amount of added sugars, chemicals, and flavors that can counteract the health benefits of yogurt," Dr. Haver told me. "Plain Greek yogurt is a better source of probiotics and protein. My favorite additions are berries, chia seeds, ground flax, and hemp seeds for added nutrients and flavor. Other sources of foods rich in probiotics are kimchi, kombucha, miso, Chinese pickles, and fermented cheeses like feta. If you can't tolerate dairy and you're really struggling to enjoy probiotic rich foods, don't despair; there are some good studies looking at probiotic supplements for women in menopause. I always say try to get your nutrients from food first."

I've heard a lot about intermittent fasting, where you try to have a certain number of hours not eating, so, for example, you fit all your food intake into an eight- or ten-hour window (say, having breakfast at 10:00 a.m. and dinner over by 6:00 p.m.).

Dr. Haver is for it: "I've been a fan of intermittent fasting for a long time for the anti-inflammatory benefits. I have, with age, adjusted my eating window to include more time for me to be able to incorporate my increased protein goals of 100 to 120 grams per day."

There was a time not long ago when doctors tended to measure whether you were a healthy weight using the body mass index, or BMI, which is calculated by dividing your weight in kilograms by your height in meters squared, or your weight in pounds divided by your height in inches squared times 703. A "normal" weight in this system is 18.5 to 24.9. (I don't use scales myself. I monitor my weight by noticing which pairs of my jeans fit.)

In 2023, the American Medical Association voted to stop relying on the BMI as a primary way of assessing weight and health. Many doctors now recommend that menopausal women use a waist-to-hip ratio, or WHR, to assess risk factors for cardiometabolic disease.

"Every woman should know this number," says Dr. Haver. (But

in my experience, most women don't know theirs. When I first heard Dr. Haver say this, I didn't know mine!)

Here's how you find it: Divide your waist circumference by your hip circumference. This is your WHR. If it's 0.8 or lower, you have a lower risk for things like heart disease, stroke, cancer, and type 2 diabetes. If it's 0.86 or higher, you have a higher risk.

This can be a good measurement to take at home, as I know that going to the doctor's office and getting undressed and onto the scale can sometimes be triggering or humiliating. And seeing this number change can be an early predictor of changes to your health. Waist-to-hip ratio often rises in menopause, and it can be connected to a higher likelihood of hip fractures, some cancers, and heart disease. But the good news is that with diet and exercise you can get that number down, and that will lower your risk for those problems.

Another thing doctors advise us to keep an eye on at this age: alcohol intake. Alcohol can change how the body metabolizes estrogen, and it can contribute to liver problems, heart disease, and osteoporosis. The Centers for Disease Control and Prevention advises that women not have more than one alcoholic drink per day. Chardonnay used to be a good friend, and now it's turned on us like a robber's dog.

And of course now, adding to the noise about what to eat or drink or not, there are new weight-loss drugs like Ozempic and Mounjaro. I'm told that if someone has intractable weight problems that are jeopardizing their health (more than just an extra ten or fifteen pounds), it could make sense for them to take these drugs to get down to a weight that is healthier. But if the drugs cause you to lose your appetite, then you have to make sure that you're still getting the nutrients you need from whatever it is you are able to make yourself eat.

Just to be clear: I'm not endorsing these weight-loss drugs personally. I've seen friends find great success with them and also friends who have gone too far with their weight loss, to the point of concern. And I worry about long-term effects since we don't have decades of research on them yet. That said, doctors are becoming increasingly knowledgeable about these drugs as they become more widely used.

Dr. Haver says before she prescribes these drugs, she will start a menopausal woman with elevated visceral fat (she has an electrical impedance scanner in her office that measures muscle mass and visceral fat) on HRT and a nutrition plan for three months. Afterward, she will reassess the patient's progress and visceral fat loss. If the patient continues to struggle, they then discuss adding in something like Ozempic. "These drugs are dramatically improving the health and quality of life of some of my patients. Some who have been on the diet cycle for decades may find that this is the only thing that works."

Still, there are risks. Dr. Haver has patients on these drugs return at least every six weeks for a body scan to track their muscle mass and fat loss. (She notes that obese patients very rarely have muscle mass issues because they've been carrying around the equivalent of weighted blankets every day, and so their muscles are strong.)

Menopocalypse author and women's health and fitness expert Amanda Thebe says she understands why women might feel overwhelmed by nutrition advice at this age. "It is so difficult to know which way to turn, especially if you get your nutritional advice from social media," she said. "Quick tip: don't! *Carbs are bad. No, hang on—meat is bad. No, we need more plants. But plants contain lectins, which are bad, too. Maybe we just eat fat. I'll go full keto, only I have high cholesterol and need to reduce my saturated fat. . . .* It's a bloody nightmare, and I don't blame women for trying enticing diets targeted to our pain points during menopause."

From what nutrition doctors have told me, it's best to keep things simple and focus on the bedrocks of nutrition. Then we're able to make choices that suit us, our goals, and how our bodies respond to food.

**Things They Really Should Tell Us
About a Menopausal Diet**

- Menopause requires us to eat differently. Women at this stage in life should be eating more protein. Try to eat less added sugar. Cut out soda, sweetened juice, and flavored yogurt. Try to get a lot of fiber.
- Drink alcohol only in moderation—if at all.
- Calculate your waist-to-hip ratio. Forget about BMI. Think "strong," not "thin."
- Consider intermittent fasting.

Amanda Thebe's Nutrition Primer

There are three macronutrients: carbohydrates, protein, and fats. "Macro" simply means "large." These foods contain micronutrients ("small"): vitamins and minerals that are compounds essential for bodily functions. The three macronutrients have different functions in the body.

- **CARBOHYDRATES:** Despite our being made to fear carbs, they are the body's preferred fuel. Carbs when eaten are broken down into simple sugars, glucose and fructose, and the body just loves them to give us energy. Glucose even crosses the blood-brain barrier, which can be helpful for clearing brain fog and lifting chronic fatigue. All carbs are sugars, but we should look at them on a spectrum, because not all carbs are created equal. Carbs come in two categories, complex and simple.
  - Complex carbs, like sweet potatoes or whole grains, contain more than one sugar, whereas simple carbs contain just one. Complex carbs take longer for the body to break down than simple sugars do and usually contain an abundance of fiber or starch, as well

as water and micronutrients. They're good for your overall health, especially your gut health, and really shouldn't be avoided.

- My advice regarding simple sugars is to keep them to a minimum. The current recommended guideline for added sugars is no more than 25 grams per day, because too much sugar directly correlates to increased disease risk. Added sugar typically has very little nutrient value and is high in calories, but it usually tastes pretty good. Omitting sugars from your diet completely will usually make you want to binge on them later, so limit the amount of candy, soda, and delicious baked goods you consume to the occasional treat.

- **PROTEIN:** I love talking about protein because we really do need it as we age, and particularly through menopause. In order to hang on to the muscle we have and even build more, the body utilizes a process called "muscle protein synthesis" (MPS). This is essentially taking the protein you eat, breaking it down into amino acids, and using it as a stimulus to build, repair, and grow muscles. Estrogen is a key player in MPS, so when it starts to decline in menopause, you need to make sure that you are helping this system along by eating adequate protein. The current recommendation is 0.8 grams of protein per kilogram of bodyweight per day. But for ease I often tell menopausal women to try to eat 100 grams of protein per day. Protein also keeps big sugar surges at bay, so when you feel that 2:00 p.m. slump, reach for the roast turkey rather than a blueberry muffin!

- **FATS:** I think everybody knows by now that a diet rich in saturated fats increases risk for cardiovascular disease, which is a real pity, because my favorite food group is butter! But most menopausal women of our generation have a fear of fats, which probably stems from the low-fat/fat-free 1990s. Do you remember standing in the supermarket when all those sleazy magazines promoted low-fat grapefruit diets? It's hard to shake off those diet tropes. The fact is that fats are actually important in our diet. They are an energy source. Fat helps the body absorb some vitamins and minerals and is utilized in a number of body functions, including improved immunity.

- Unsaturated fats protect the heart and improve immunity. The current guidelines suggest that 20 to 35 percent of your diet should be made up of healthy fats, such as olive oil, vegetable oils, fatty fish (like salmon and tuna), avocados, nuts, and seeds. This would mean a 2,000-calories-per-day diet should include approximately 500 calories, or 56 grams, of fat.
- Saturated fats—which usually come from animals (like butter, meat, and milk) but also from tropical plant sources (like coconut and palm oils)—should definitely be limited.

The best menopause diet advice you can follow is to eat a balanced diet that consists of lots of complex carbs, especially from plant sources, with enough protein to support your body, and a side of healthy fats.

Dr. Mary Claire Haver's Personal Supplement Cabinet

FIBER: If needed, I take extra fiber to reach a total 35 grams a day. To obtain this goal, I enjoy a daily avocado, and while I eat meat, my diet is heavily plant based.

MAGNESIUM: Many of us are deficient in magnesium. There are various types of this mineral; I take one called NeuroMag (its generic name is magnesium L-threonate). This formulation reliably crosses the blood-brain barrier. I take it in the afternoon and have found it helps me stay calm in the evening and aids in my sleep. I often recommend it to my patients for the same reason.

VITAMIN D: Most of my patients are vitamin D deficient, and I have struggled with this as well. I created a vitamin D supplement that contains 4,000 IU of vitamin D, vitamin K for increased absorption, and omega-3 fatty acids for the anti-inflammatory benefits.

OMEGA-3 FATTY ACIDS: I take a combo of omega-3 and vitamin D.

COLLAGEN: Collagen has been shown to improve bone density in women with osteoporosis and osteopenia, a warning sign of osteoporosis. It can also improve joint health and skin elasticity.

CHAPTER FOURTEEN

WORKING IT OUT

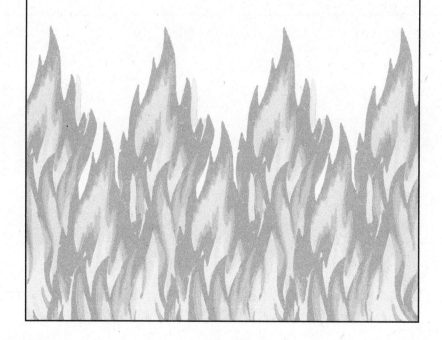

In Hollywood, of course, you are so often being looked at. There can be pressure to stay slim and to fight the effects of aging as much as possible. I've found the best approach to this preoccupation is to look for the humor in others' ideas about what your body should be. (After a night shoot, as we finished up at 5:00 a.m., I caught a glimpse of myself upside down in a mirrored table; I swear I looked like Nick Nolte.) It's worth asking as we move through our days and worry about how we look: Who is our perceived audience, and why do we care so much about what that person thinks?

Friends of mine often criticize their aging bodies, particularly areas I guarantee no one else is paying any attention to. One recently said, "The skin between the creases in my neck is beginning to look a bit like an overstretched band of elastic." She pointed to her neck, and I honestly had no idea what she meant. I thought her neck looked great!

I find it's hard to tune out this noise in my own head sometimes, too. Maybe that's why as part of my regular routine I like to take loud dance classes in a dark room. Less than five minutes in, I'm having the time of my life. (I especially like it when the dance sequences are short enough that I don't get confused!)

Being there as a middle-aged woman now, I feel grateful to be alive and still able to do most of the things that I used to be able to do. And yes, I do them more carefully. In the past, high-impact exercise has exacerbated my recurring back issues, so I don't do all the crazy jumping like the young girls in the front. I'm happy in the back, and I avoid the jerky movements that might tweak my frozen shoulder. But I love to feel my body come alive.

The women I like to exercise with are happy to be in the room. They are not only there for leaner limbs or muscled arms, but as much as to become strong, they are there for the celebration of life and the affirmation that we can still keep moving our bodies in sync with the music. We made an appointment, we broke away from the household, and we did it for ourselves. We showed up, and we had a blast. I find it cleansing and cathartic. Being in the room filled with lots of sweating ladies is both fun and meaningful, such a good release and a necessary comfort, even if we have to reach for the earplugs.

Doctors recommend a certain amount of cardio exercise during menopause for improved mental health, better sleep, and overall fitness, especially because in middle age we tend to gain weight around the middle, which is a risk factor for heart disease. I feel like it's so much easier to exercise when it's fun and when you feel comfortable wherever you choose to work out.

In the past I went to exercise classes out of a desire to look better—as a friend likes to say, "not for inner peace but for outer hotness." I was vain and too conscious of others' opinions. In midlife, if we are lucky and also honest with ourselves, I think it's possible to lose our competitiveness with other women and support one another. We can celebrate everyone's achievements. When people ask me how to get this confidence, I tell them the only way I know of is to live long enough. If you're fortunate to make it to midlife, you realize that no one's looking at you as harshly as you look at yourself. Everyone else is absorbed in their own dramas and insecurities. If it all feels too hard: Fake it till you make it! Retrain the thinking!

My friend and I walked out of a class the other day on cloud nine. It was like we'd gone back to the clubs, with the dark room and the disco lights, and current music mixed with some good oldies. We felt invigorated.

That was a good reminder that I need to work out for my mental health, too. If I drop my routine, which I often do, I feel crappy. So even when I'm staying in a hotel or an Airbnb, I still try to do a workout. I'm not fanatical like I used to be. I used to be a five-day-a-week person. Now I try to exercise two or three times a week.

I know exercise classes aren't for everyone. Some people stay fit by walking or swimming or lifting weights in their garage. A lot of women our age respond well to Pilates, which increases both strength and flexibility. What the experts seem to agree on is that we just have to do *something*.

To avoid losing muscle mass and gaining weight, the majority of menopausal women need both aerobic activity and strength training. Weight gain can be connected not just to what and how you're eating but also to how much you're sleeping, how you're genetically coded, and whether or not you're depressed.

Strength training is also important in midlife for bone health, which prevents muscle loss.

Amanda Thebe told me, "We know that we are at an increased risk of fracture and osteoporosis, 'the silent thief,' after menopause. Strength training at all ages is the best way to prevent bone loss, and at menopause it is the best way to prevent further loss. When you do strength training and create an overload on your muscles, you encourage bone growth."

Dr. Mary Claire Haver said that women should shift their ideal from thin to strong. Agreed. Thinness isn't a measure of health. Becoming stronger also helps us maintain our balance and decreases our risk of falls and fractures with age.

"When we look at female longevity, we are living longer than men, but we live 20 percent of that life in poorer health than those male counterparts," said Dr. Haver. "If I'm going to have the extra years, I want to be like Queen Elizabeth. She had some advantages, of course—probably the world's best medical care—but she met with the prime minister and then went and took a nap and died. I don't want that long, protracted area of my life where I'm going to need long-term care. And so that's going to depend on me staying strong over skinny, watching nutrition over calories, and doing things to keep my brain healthy. My hormone therapy is a part of this strategy too."

Amanda Thebe agrees. "Often the conversation in the menopause world is very binary, and we don't see a space where menopause hormone therapy and exercise can coexist," she told me. "I often hear comments like 'Exercise will replace my missing hormones' or 'I'm taking testosterone to stay strong.' Exercise doesn't replace your missing hormones, and the doses of hormones, particularly testosterone, prescribed to women are so nominal that they don't impact strength training in any meaningful way. These are all soundbites that quite simply need to stop. Medications do not replace exercise, and exercise does not replace hormone therapy. All have positive effects and should be viewed through that lens. There is no one-point solution for menopause."

Thebe continued, "If you are at high risk of osteoporosis, estrogen plays an important role in preventing bone loss and reducing the risk for fractures and joint pain, and it offers some protective benefit to the heart. These positives are stated by the Menopause Society and should give those women who take HRT a sense of relief. The problem occurs when the benefits of HRT are presented to women as a 'magic pill' that will help them live forever and be a cure for all ails. When the facts presented are bent to produce a biased narrative, the people who suffer are those trying to make an informed choice. Whether or not you choose to take HRT—or any other medication for that matter—you should *definitely* be looking at ways to improve your daily movement and consider starting strength training."

My own regimen has settled into something manageable, but it took a while to get here. I bounced around from every workout known to man. Not only do exercise fads change like denim trends, but I also get bored easily, and my body tells me when it's time to change things up. In my twenties, I was jogging and doing Ashtanga, a highly disciplined type of yoga. In both pursuits, I was probably chasing some center or balance in my life. In my thirties, I continued to run miles and miles, like I was trying to beat the clock. In my forties, I was doing boot camp classes, as though I were working through rage. Now, seeking flexibility, focus, and strength in my fifties, I've gotten into weight training, dance classes, and as much stretching as I can stand to create clarity, strength, and fun.

One recent afternoon, my friend and I went to a yoga class together in our crop tops. As the class began, I realized that we were the oldest people in the room by at least fifteen years. While I moved through the poses, I cast my mind back to when I was in my twenties, the age of a lot of the other women there. Back then I felt so at odds with my body that I covered myself up with plenty of literal clothing and metaphorical armor.

Those days are over. Our bodies aren't as taut or injury-free or unlined as they were twenty or thirty years ago. I've given birth and spent decades in all weathers, and it shows. One of my girlfriends has nicknamed my stomach Benjamin Button. It's so wrinkled that it resembles a paper bag that's been twisted up and left damp on the side of the road. And yet, I'll wear a crop top now, which I never would have done back before I had the paper-bag stomach.

I'm proud of what my body's endured. I'll show it to the world if I want to. At this age, we can exercise not just for vanity but for joy and health, which feels much more rewarding.

I'm not sure if the younger women at that class noticed us at all. If they did, perhaps they thought of us as crusty old ladies. But I'd like to think they saw us, joking with each other and smiling, happy in our fifties bodies, and thought that maybe getting older wouldn't be so bad. I am aging, and it's a privilege. What's the alternative?

Simple Strength Training Exercises You Could Do Right Now

For times when I'm unable to get to the gym, I'm a fan of the Scientific 7-Minute Workout *The New York Times* published a while back. It's great when you're traveling and have only a few minutes to spare. Here's a version that I do often:

1. 20 squats (Do them like you're sitting down in a chair.)
2. 20 lunges (You can start out just taking a small step forward and build up to a broader range of motion as you get in the habit.)

3. 20-second plank (I have one friend who, in the course of a summer, worked her way up from being able to hold a plank for ten seconds to three minutes!)
4. 20 push-ups (While you're in a plank, might as well do some of these.)
5. 20 dead lifts with hand weights. (Good to have hand weights around your desk for when you're bored! And if you don't have any, you can just put your hands behind your back, fingers facing forward and resting on a chair or table, then push yourself up and down 20 times.)

Frozen Shoulder Release Stretches

- Stand with your frozen shoulder against a wall. Keep that hand flat against the wall as if you're washing a car and do a full rotation of the hand on the wall in a circle. Do clockwise and then switch directions.

- Do a plank on your forearms. Move your body forward and back over your arms.

- Use an elastic band or towel and hold at each end. Lift it from wheelbarrow position to over your head. Then do the same from behind your back and lift in tiny pulses. Then try it gently on the diagonal in front and behind your back.

- For more frozen shoulder exercises, google dumbbell halos, scapular push-ups (elbows locked), thoracic stretching, finger walks on a wall, floor slides in hip bridge, assisted shoulder flexion, and lateral stretches.

CHAPTER FIFTEEN

WHAT DOES "FAMILY" LOOK LIKE NOW?

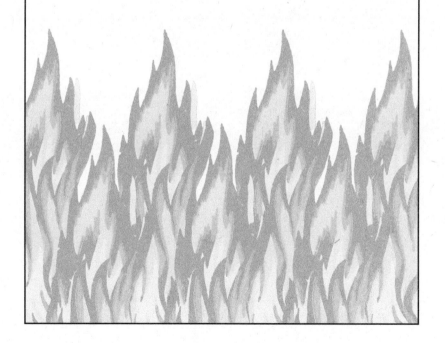

"The experience of menopause is not limited to physio-logical symptoms and 'bad moods.' It is also a time of truth-telling," one friend said to me by email.

It's not a coincidence that many marriages end around midlife. In the absence of the intoxication of raising young children and/or the distractions of career building, we attempt to settle into a new quiet. For me, that developing solitude revealed a long-muted voice inside that I could no longer ignore, and I began to understand that my marriage was over.

Statistically, I could live another thirty or forty years and not be an outlier. Would I limp to the finish line with someone I had grown apart from just because we had fallen in love at twenty-two? The combination of an empty nest and my expired womb became a drumbeat of freedom. Toleration was yesterday's theme. Today I was reborn and optimistic about my new chapter alone. Maybe not yet repaired or redeemed, but healing would come.

I packed a bag and told my family I was taking a gap year, thrilled to be alone on my new adventure. It didn't last long; within twelve months, I had fallen deeply in love with my new partner, and I hope I will be with him for the rest of my life. But had I not found him, I know I would not have regretted my deci-sion; I had made the choice on my own terms. Finally a grown-up, at fifty-two years old.

I've heard many similar stories from women at this age, of completely reconfiguring their lives and rethinking their relation-ships with their partners, careers, children, friends, or themselves. So many of us are asking big questions again, or for the first time: What does it mean to be a full person in relationship to other people? To be at once a lover, a partner, a friend? Perhaps a spouse or a parent, or maybe not?

I also have so many friends who cherish their long marriages and feel that staying with the same person for decades, through various crises, allowed them to "level up" in the relationship, to reach new heights of security and closeness.

Modern Elder Academy founder and CEO Chip Conley, who's also the author of *Learning to Love Midlife,* told me, "Hopefully, by this time, we're not looking for Mr. or Ms. Perfect, because that person doesn't exist. I don't know about you, but it's too high of a standard for me. The question we should ask ourselves is not *Who is the ideal partner?* but *Who can I co-create the ideal lifestyle conditions with?*

"That helped me so much and led me back to my partner from whom I'd split sixteen years earlier, knowing that we had very comparable ideas of how we wanted to live our lives. Let's also re-alize that relationships go through cycles, so the most important coping mechanisms are communication and respect."

After my breakup with Liev, I was prepared to "date myself," as they say, indefinitely, to lean into my role as a mother and as a friend rather than into dating. But then I fell in love with Billy. After seven years with him, at the age of fifty-four, I got married for the first time.

My friends took me out for an absolutely ridiculous bachelor-ette party. Amid all the crude jokes, my best friend reminded me of what I'd said when I first fell in love with Billy: "Loving him is the kindest thing I've ever done for myself."

This relationship has made my life so much richer and eased so many burdens. For one thing, it's wonderful to have another grown-up around. For me, one of the greatest challenges of rela-tionships in menopause has been parenting teenagers. I thought being a parent when the kids were little was hard! But now I'm finding lots of new issues as they get close to moving out of the house. I've been dealing with anticipatory grief, if that's a thing. And probably they are too. So it's a big collision of grief and panic.

Teenagers want to try everything even as they cannot see two steps in front of themselves. My kids like to get away with things. They certainly aren't the type to say, "Well, it's getting late, better turn in."

As developmental psychologist Dr. Aliza Pressman told me: "Teenagers are at a moment of all gas and no brakes, changing emotions and changing hormones, and so they're going to potentially fly off the handle and not necessarily be self-regulated. Their brains aren't at capacity to be as fully self-regulated as an adult brain."

In some ways, parenting teenagers is like raising two-year-olds again. You might find yourself worrying constantly. When toddlers learn that word "no," they overuse it. It's their first glimpse of power. That repeats itself with teenagers, only it becomes a declaration of identity and independence. It's still a power move: "No, that's not how you do it! Leave me alone." They always know better!

Only instead of fear that they're going to fall into the pool or down the stairs, I fret that they're getting into cars with friends who are brand-new drivers. When my son's friends come over, I find myself staring them in the eye to gauge if they're sober and responsible. If they're about to get behind the wheel, I am always tempted to test their eye-hand coordination.

The worry is only one part of it. The day-to-day work of raising children that has consumed me for the past two decades is almost over. They're all too ready for a break from me. Yet, on my side, this transition feels abrupt and almost cruel. The first time I got that "What are you still doing here?" look as they shut the door to their room, I thought, *I'm not ready!* I felt like I was failing some kind of test of psychological growth, incapable of absorbing this new reality with expansiveness. I was *sad*. And I found the knowledge that this was how it was going to be for the next few years truly heartbreaking.

At each juncture in life, we are thrown challenges that force us to learn and grow. But this one—*Congratulations! Your kids are done with you! And at the exact moment when you are no longer physically capable of ever bearing more of them!*—has been one of those blows that has resulted in a new form of grief. Of course you want them to make their own way in the world. That doesn't take away from how melancholy it feels, though, when their friends pick them up and they run off without so much as a glance back.

I've been asking my friends how they feel about the approaching an empty nest.

One told me she's focused on giving her children the tools they require not to need her. Among her advice: "Go enjoy life—sex, drugs, rock 'n' roll—but if you smoke cigarettes or get a tattoo I'll break your legs." (I think she's confident they have no interest in drugs.)

"I'll be honest, it makes me super sad to think about," one friend said. "My cousin and I talk about it often. Sometimes it helps us to imagine that when our kids are gone we will re-create a time we shared together in our early twenties baking, partying, talking, and making terrible decisions about men. Other times it helps us to imagine ourselves living together in an assisted-living facility dancing with our walkers and eating Jell-O with our dentures. We send one another memes of old women walking, dancing, and sitting on rockers together. My other friend and I have plans to take walking trips in England and Ireland, as we have decided that older women with empty nests need to walk a lot."

Midlife can often bring intense caregiving responsibilities, whether for kids we had late or for aging parents. It's so often in families that the hardest jobs fall on the middle-aged women. According to the Family Caregiver Alliance, about two-thirds of caregiving—whether for elderly parents or a sibling or children (and so often more than one of these simultaneously!)—is done by women.

One friend told me: "I have had the lion's share of responsibility with care for my father when he was dying of cancer and care for my mother throughout the years. It can be challenging to care for an elderly parent and kids at the same time. I can feel like my mother is my fourth child. At times I'll try and plan something to please all three of my kids and then she'll pipe in that she'd rather do something else. I'll think, *I can't put one more person's needs, desires, and moods above my own, or I'll drown!*"

It helps to look at the upside of times when our caregiving role lessens, as when the children leave the house. You'll have more time for yourself, your partner, and your career. You are done taking care of others; now is the time to do things for yourself!

Then comes our reckoning with how much we have sacrificed of ourselves to others over the years.

Eve Rodsky, author of *Fair Play*, calls attention to the damage done to women by the unequal division of labor: "Women are making more money as breadwinners, while also doing more unpaid cognitive labor (often called the 'mental load'). As a result, they are growing sicker mentally and physically."

She says the unfairness of so many households can even exacerbate menopause symptoms. "We don't talk enough about this: if you don't have the time to be well because your time has been hijacked by other people and by your roles as parent, partner, professional, then menopause is going to be worse." She's identified two thousand examples of unpaid labor that women do more than men. The only exception: taking out the garbage gets split fifty-fifty.

Rodsky hit a wall in her own marriage when her kids were little. She was driving to pick up her toddler from preschool, her breast pump in her bag and a client's mediation contract in her lap. Her husband texted: "I'm surprised you didn't get blueberries."

Understandably, she snapped. Eventually, she was able to articulate to her husband what she was feeling and what she saw as the solution. I think it's a good script for us all to consider when we find ourselves doing too much for others without receiving support in return:

There are twenty-four hours in my day just like yours. It's not going to be judged by money anymore. Or whether you believe that somehow your time is more valuable because you earn more.

In our household, we both get twenty-four hours in a day. I'm only going to be in this relationship if you value my time as equal to your time. It doesn't have to necessarily look completely equal in unpaid labor, but we both have to find a balance that feels fair. And we are going to find equality in our leisure time. To start, you'll take Saturdays, and I'll take Sundays while we figure this shit out. Until then, I am not available on Sundays. And I don't care whether you call it a "spa day" or try to guilt me. That's not going to work anymore. I'll do whatever I want to do.

"When we asked women how they felt about midlife, the two words that were the biggest in the word cloud were 'overwhelm' and 'boredom.' That was very depressing to me because if you're overwhelmed, you should not be bored! We realized that women didn't feel as if they had permission to be unavailable for even a moment. Women are just conditioned to anticipate other people's discomfort," said Rodsky. "Once I understood that distinction, then I could have empathy with others' discomfort, but it wasn't infecting my decision making."

In all of this work, it's helpful to be honest with your family and to have people around you who are willing to speak openly about menopause, the empty nest, and what all of it means for us. I'm lucky in that regard. I credit that to Billy, a forward-thinking man who'd done a load of therapy before I met him.

Unfortunately, I feel like a huge proportion of the male population gets squeamish or scared around this stuff. Mood swings and the stresses of this time of life can make it difficult to parse why we're feeling sad or off. Friends or partners might not react well to our emotional intensity combined with a lack of clarity. I've seen friends' male partners who got defensive in ways that were unhelpful, or who saw their partners' challenges as nuisances or things that didn't concern them at all.

One friend of mine reports: "Steve asked me how long menopause lasts. I asked him why. He said, 'I want to know when we can turn off the air-conditioning.'"

One of my most popular Instagram posts was a video I took of my friend Ursula responding to her husband's question, "What time's dinner?" She did a hilarious little dance in which she flipped him off with both hands. The reaction to that post spoke to the exasperation so many women feel when it falls to them to carry more than their fair share of the work that goes into running a household. So how can we advocate for ourselves? And what should we even be asking for in a relationship?

Dr. Pressman told me that in midlife we should focus not necessarily on having romance (though she's said we should certainly feel free to enjoy that too!), but rather on establishing at least one loving relationship, whether that's with a partner or with a friend: "Women thrive when they have at least one human in their life who will tell them lovingly that there's broccoli in their teeth. It's not about a romantic partner. It really is about quality connections."

The Harvard Study of Adult Development has shown that deep relationships are huge factors in a person's quality of life and even in their longevity.

Dr. Pressman is known in the parenting world for defining the key principles that build resilience in children, but in our conversation I realized that they apply beautifully to all our intimate connections. Her five Rs are relationship, reflection, regulation, repair, and rules. Here's how she described them to me in a recent meeting:

RELATIONSHIP is exactly what it sounds like: feeling connected to and seeing another person. I think the most heartening lesson from relationship research is that it takes only one caregiver for us to build resilience. It could be a coach, or a teacher, or a friend, or a partner. The presence of that one person with whom you feel safe and seen and connected can buffer the impact of toxic stress. I think the fact that we can do all of that just by being in a relationship is so refreshing in this world where we have so little control.

REFLECTION is taking time to pause and make intentional choices. We can do that by thinking back to how we first experienced love and what that experience means for how we want to give love to our kids and to our partners as well as how we're able to receive love. When you think this way, you don't respond reactively. This change in perspective allows us to change patterns in our lives in ways that feel right for us.

REGULATION is both co-regulation and self-regulation. It's a combination of not blowing up at the barista who gets the order wrong and being able to distinguish between real and imagined threats. The prefrontal cortex is not fully available in developing brains. Its growth isn't complete until between age eighteen and the later twenties. Before that age, you'll need to borrow the nervous system of someone more mature to learn the best way to regulate yourself. Studies, particularly with mothers and children, show that the more self-regulated the mother is, the more self-regulated the child is.

REPAIR becomes necessary because it's hard to regulate oneself in every situation. Nobody's going to get it right all the time, and if they did, it *wouldn't* be right; it would be a disservice to their relationships. This is because without discord, you can't have repair. And when you don't repair, you don't learn that discord is not the end of the universe.

If there was just discord, the relationship wouldn't be healthy. But when you disconnect, you can come back to connection. That can be zoning out and looking at your phone and then coming back together, or it can be a fight.

The fifth principle is **RULES**. Rules comprise boundaries and limits, both of which women have long felt guilty about expressing.

Isn't all that *great*? We need to have tremendous compassion for ourselves and our friends; that's why I particularly love the repair principle. Menopause is the time to lean into our relationships with our friends and our work, and also to nurture whatever else we're passionate about. My friends and I are always fantasizing about what our endgame looks like. We're constantly sending one another notices of houses for sale for a dollar in glorious locations, or incredible trips we could take together, or nursing homes where we could while away our hours playing bingo.

We have many a lunch that starts with "This just happened. Can I cry to you about it for a minute?" and that ends with "I loved seeing you. By the way, before you go back to the office: you've got something in your teeth."

How to Talk to Your Family About Menopause

Ideally, women's healthcare is just something that you talk about regularly, the same way you talk about the weather. I have a lot of friends who diligently hid their tampons from the kids and then when puberty arrived for their daughters, it called for a much longer conversation than it would have if their daughters had been exposed to the reality of menstruation all along. Similarly, it's good to talk about menopause early and often. But for those who are just getting started discussing this issue, Dr. Pressman has a suggestion for how to bring it up, not only with your children but with your partner. The key, she says, is to name it, so no one starts imagining that the tension is their fault rather than just the result of this very natural event.

Here's Her Script for Talking to Kids:

Maybe you've noticed me having a hot flash or being irritable. These are some of the changes that happen as I'm going through this transition. I want you to know, because otherwise you're not going to understand why sometimes I'm uncomfortable physically and sometimes I seem emotional. The good news is that I know how to take care of myself. You don't have to take care of me. Still,

it's important that you know what's going on so you're not imag-
ining that it's anything else happening beyond this normal pro-
cess. If you see some of these things, please remember that they
have nothing to do with you. I'm working on it, and I don't need
you to worry; my doctor is taking care of me.

And Here's a Script for Partners:

"Stay the hell away from me!" I say.

No. Don't say that. Try this version from Dr. Pressman instead,
and be prepared to listen to questions and comments at the end:

I want to tell you what's going on because I want us to have the
best relationship we can have, and I'm going to need support
when things are getting heated with our teenagers or others and
I don't feel like I'm at operating at full capacity. So please help me
out. I'm caring for myself. There are things we can do to make
this easier if we're in it together.

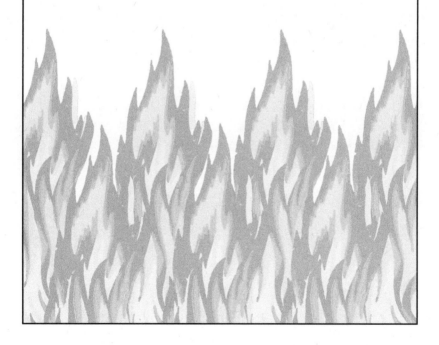

CHAPTER SIXTEEN

GETTING THE MEDICAL CARE YOU NEED

When I get sick, my husband calls me Winston Churchill, because left to my own devices, I dig in. I'll never go to the doctor for a cold. I will show up to work having slept just two hours. I am the classic English stiff-upper-lip type, bustling about while half dead, shouting, "Soldier on, for God's sake!"

I've learned from Billy, who takes good care of himself and of me, to be less stoic and kinder to my body. We shouldn't try to push through everything all the time to prove how tough we are, how self-sufficient. There's no "pushing through" menopause, a life change that affects so many aspects of our bodies and our moods. It demands attention, even if we have an easy time of it. As we've learned, perimenopause can last a decade, and the time on the other side of menopause could comprise a third to a half of our life!

I began learning about the importance of medical advocacy and how much women put up with during my first time in the labor and delivery ward. My first child's birth story is certainly not a warm and fuzzy one.

I went into it all with high hopes. My closest friend, Rebecca, is what's known as an "earth mother." She had her first baby in her midtwenties, at home in the bath, with no doctors around. And she went on to have two more children. For her third, they had to cut her jeans off her because the baby was sliding out on its own. She was ahead of every trend with mothering. I'm pretty sure she ate her own placenta in an omelet.

When I got pregnant, she was acting as a kind of doula for my coming delivery, and she coached me on doing it naturally. From everything I'd read, I was convinced that a natural birth would be best—to the point where it became something of an obsession. I thought, *I need to do this in the most authentic, natural way, the way that we've seen images of and read stories about. If I can't do it that way, then I'm less than, somehow. I must endure the pain, and I must not let my body be cut.* I was obviously "musterbating" a lot.

Mind you, my friend wasn't saying any of these things. She was just trying to help me avoid unnecessary interventions. I was imposing all these moral judgments on myself.

The original aim was for me to have the baby at home, but soon after I went into labor, I couldn't deal with the pain, and I wasn't dilating. I went to the hospital, and in the early hours of the morning, after about three hours of laboring naturally, I said, "Okay, I can't do this, forget it." I got an epidural.

My friend came the following afternoon, when I was finally close to fully dilated. She was trying to coach me to bear down, but I'd lost feeling. Everyone was saying, "Push, push, try to push!"

I felt like I was pushing so hard my head was going to explode off my body, but apparently that sensation was not being reflected in what was happening between my legs.

My friend started chatting with the doctor, who had also delivered her last baby (the one that slid out like a toboggan down a ski slope). She said, "Oh, let her have one more go, one more go!" But my baby was in distress, and the monitor was going berserk. Someone in a position of authority said, "Okay, everybody out of the way, this lady's going on the gurney and into the ER right this minute for an emergency C-section."

As you might imagine, the combination of the painkillers and Pitocin and anxiety and lack of sleep had not created a particularly spiritual labor experience. When the C-section was over, I had the shakes, and I was scared to touch my own baby. There'd been so many hands on me and the baby by this point that I felt like I had failed at being a natural mother.

Postpartum, I had some residual feelings of inadequacy. I was unsure of how to navigate the coming weeks. Then there was the mass exodus of hormones. And seeing this big gash in my body, I started sobbing.

I'll never forget how, in the maternity ward, women were looking down at their bodies, brutalized by labor or surgery—and still taking notes as they were taught how to breastfeed while simultaneously being gracious to guests. All the women in that ward looking shell-shocked as their milk was coming in, or wasn't, and thinking, *Oh my God, my body! What just happened?* Sometimes one of us would cry without even knowing quite why—which speaks to hormones being such powerful forces. Nothing in my life has ever felt quite so extraordinary as the experience of giving birth.

I think it's most helpful to think of menopausal changes as part of the larger question of how to take care of ourselves through the many transformations women go through over the course of a lifetime. Dr. Mary Claire Haver advised me to "view health and healthcare as a toolkit, encompassing nutrition, physical activity, stress management, sleep optimization, pharmaceutical options, and community support. Enjoy the present moments and relationships. Acknowledge life's inevitable challenges, including family losses and natural disasters. In the midst of balancing everything, prioritize self-care for mental, emotional, and physical health. Menopause is inevitable, and preparation is essential."

It might take a willingness to be seen as bossy to make it comfortably through this stage of life. Women's bodies endure a lot. If we're complaining of discomfort, our doctor should be attending to us rather than shrugging it off. Advocating for yourself can be hard, especially when you've received a lifetime of indoctrination that women should suck it up and be pleasing. Also, doctors' visits are stressful! I can't tell you how many women I've talked to who've gone to their annual exams ready to finally get help and the second they're on the table forget everything they wanted to say, even if it's just the one question: "I've been reading about menopause. Could we discuss HRT?"

"You would think 'I'd like to discuss it,' wouldn't be hard to say, but of course it is," Dr. Carol Tavris told me. "The history of women's experience with menopause is you didn't talk about it. It made you feel old. There was a stigma associated with it. You might say something to your friends, or tell funny stories about your miserable hot flashes, but you didn't seek information. Women today are more outspoken and more demanding. They want answers and information and are not ashamed to be going through menopause. And as women are learning that they were misled about hormones, they are getting mad. Avrum [Bluming] and I get messages like these every day: *I'm so angry that I went off HRT for ten years. I'm so angry that my doctor won't prescribe hormones for me. I'm so angry that my doctor won't listen to me.* So the most important message for women going through menopause today is this: Demand that you and your doctor have a partnership. It's your body, your health, your well-being, and your symptoms. You are entitled to the best information and the best medical practice."

As women become more assertive with their medical teams, doctors are being pushed to be more proactive about treatment. I'm happy to see that things have changed for the better even since I went through my frustrating experience with doctors during early menopause.

Dr. Suzanne Gilberg-Lenz told me that there's been a shift in how women are approaching their midlife health. "I'm having a lot of people coming in much younger, which is great. They're saying: 'I want to get on top of this.'"

There are already plenty of health issues to keep an eye on during midlife. According to AARP, some of the most common problems in our fifties are high blood pressure, high cholesterol, arthritis, osteoporosis, cancer, anxiety, and depression.

The American Cancer Society recommends that women with an average risk for colon cancer get screened for it every ten years starting at age forty-five. And the CDC suggests getting the shingles vaccine in two doses a few months apart once you hit fifty. I wish I'd gotten it, because I recently came down with a case myself. Mercifully, I caught it early, and with medication it healed quickly.

Watching out for osteoporosis is also crucial. Especially if your parents were frail and had falls, it's worth getting a DXA scan (a bone density test) to look at your bone, fat, and muscle composition.

You lie on a flat table, and a machine goes over you for a few passes taking X-rays. It takes about twelve minutes. This is something I've been meaning to do even though I hate MRI scans ever since I had them for my migraines. They make me anxious! But I plan on doing this one and a brain scan because of Dr. Lisa Mosconi's research.

It's important for us to have the information we need to be aware of what to worry about and what not to. Heart disease is the number-one killer of women, and yet we tend to worry more about cancer than about heart disease, because breast cancer feels more frightening and it's high in the public's awareness. The good news, Dr. Avrum Bluming told me, is that "of the many thousands of women who develop any form of breast cancer, approximately 90 percent are disease-free after five years, and for some whose initial breast cancer was localized—which is the vast majority of cases—98 percent are disease-free after five years."

What else should concern us? Dr. Stacy Lindau told me, "Especially for women who have a prior cancer history, deep pain with sex—not pain that happens around the opening, but deep pain—is a symptom that should not be ignored. Bleeding after menopause is a symptom that absolutely should not be ignored. Both of those should be evaluated with a transvaginal ultrasound and possibly an endometrial biopsy as well."

When I had bleeding after menopause, I was told that the vast majority of the time the cause will prove to be something minor and treatable but that I was right to bring it up because either post-menopause bleeding or deep pain can be an indication of uterine cancer.

Dutifully, I went and got my ultrasound and biopsy. The scan found thickening of the uterine wall but nothing alarming. The doctor told me that the bleeding was likely happening because I'd just changed my dosage of estrogen and gone from the pill to the gel. And eventually it stopped. I was relieved that I'd gotten it checked out and that my concerns were taken seriously.

Dr. Sharon Malone said: "I am hopeful that the next generation of women will be less tolerant of the status quo in women's health, and are ready to shout, not whisper, 'We're not having it. So you need to go figure that out.' That is the impetus behind the advocacy work I'm doing now. I want a grassroots movement to catch fire so women can learn how to advocate for themselves. I just want women to understand what their options are and how to exercise them. I want them to have the best science-backed information available so they can make the decisions that are right for them. That's all I ask. And I know that when women get good information, they are more than capable of making good choices."

I will say that finding the right doctor is not easy, especially given the limits of insurance and scheduling, but once you get a doctor you can have a real conversation with, it's a game changer.

A Script for Talking to Your Doctor

Dr. Somi Javaid told me, "So many people ask me, 'How do I get my doctor to listen?' This is what I will say: Most doctors, including myself, go out with the best of intentions. We are working in a very, very broken healthcare system.

"A clinician is expected to finish in an eight-hour day what actually takes a human being north of twenty-seven hours to complete. So, when people say, 'Why didn't my doctor call me back? Why didn't they look up the labs? Why can't they just do it over the phone? Why didn't they call my oncologist?' Remember, they're seeing patients every seven to fifteen minutes.

"If you think about it, in gynecology we also have to let you get undressed, try to step out of the room to give you a semblance of modesty, examine you, and then enter your details into the computer and send off orders. It is an impossible task. We've set ourselves up for failure. It's why doctors are leaving the field in droves.

"We are going to have a massive shortage of ob-gyns just as we have a record number of women entering menopause. So, I tell patients, 'Your current provider may not be trained or they may not be in a system that allows them to practice the medicine that they want to practice. You have to go to someone who has the expertise and the time.'"

One way to find a menopause practitioner aside from asking your primary care doctor and your insurance company is to go to the website of the Menopause Society (menopause.org) and search by zip code.

Once you have a doctor who's listening, that's the moment to advocate for yourself. And I know you always hear "Be your own advocate," but that's easier said than done. You've heard my story in this book. I did some things right, and plenty wrong. But I finally know how to get my needs met by walking in prepared. Here's what I learned about how to talk to doctors: Don't waste time. Show up prepared with information about your body and with questions. These are a few things to jot down before you see the doctor:

1. How Things Are Going Down There

If your period has stopped, note any changes in discharge, moisture, odor, or sensation. If you're still getting a period, do all that initial noting and also track your periods in the months leading up to your annual exam via an app or on your calendar. Have a printout of that data in hand.

Dr. Kelly Casperson says to ask yourself "Do you notice, about ten days in, you start to have mini-PMS at ovulation? Or did your PMS used to be two days and now it's fourteen days? Or now you're skipping your period and it's a sixty-day-long cycle and you feel like you're PMSing for forty days of it?"

Ideally, you've noticed patterns that you can share. ("I bawl all day the day before my period." "I break things the week before my period." "My last period was in April. Since then I've only had a few days of spotting.")

2. Have You Received Any New Test Results?

Know when your last mammogram and Pap smear were and what the results were, and have on hand any blood test results that you have questions about.

3. Any Discomfort or Curious Symptoms?

Share any symptoms you're having, even if you're not sure they're gynecological. Do you have night sweats, headaches, bloating, mood swings, dry skin . . . ?

4. Sexual Health

Describe any sexual concerns you have. Are you experiencing pain during sex? A libido higher or lower than you'd like?

5. Birth Control

What birth control are you on if you're sexually active and still menstruating? Yes, fertility drops significantly starting around thirty-five, and the chance of a natural pregnancy in your forties is low, but it's not zero.

6. Diet and Medication

List any vitamins, supplements, and medications you're taking, and how you might like to drop from, change, or add to that list. If you'd like more information on HRT, say, "I've been doing some reading about hormone therapy, and I'd like to ask if you think it could help me with . . ."

Red Flags

Finally, here are some signs that you might need to find a new doctor:

1. They don't give you even the ten minutes it would take to get through the basic questions.
2. They're treating you in a dismissive manner or asking you to prove you are suffering enough to deserve treatment.
3. They say hormones are dangerous (which suggests they're not keeping up on Menopause Society guidelines). It might help to refer them to *The New York Times Magazine* story about hormones, but if it doesn't, find someone else!

CHAPTER SEVENTEEN

CLOSER TO FINE

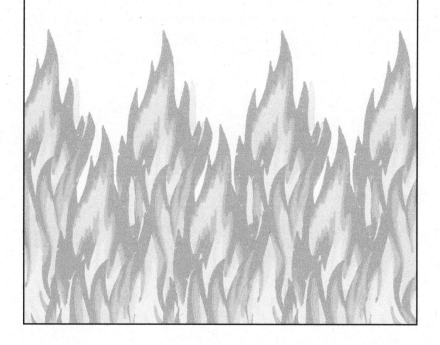

"There are years that ask questions and years that answer," said Zora Neale Hurston. My friends and I have all had years of confidence and years of confusion, years of being sure of our paths and years of having no idea what the next step is.

Midlife can be a very hard time. Plenty of us are losing parents, facing issues with our kids, or struggling in our relationships (or alone). All these things are hard enough without being barraged by physical and emotional symptoms. I hope this book will be of help for anyone trying to get a hold on this phase of life and make it a time of liberation rather than purely a time of trial. In menopause, so much has become clearer to me about my priorities and goals. I'm lucky to have two living grandmothers. One is 101 and the other is ninety-nine. So God willing I could be just over halfway through my life at this point; what a lot left to enjoy. Fingers crossed!

"There's a general peace that comes with being on the other side of it and knowing that the symptoms have calmed down," Mariella Frostrup said when I asked her about what we have to look forward to. "That, and being surrounded by the women that you've got years and years of history with. Female friendships really become a superpower when you get to this age. We need to tell our daughters this so that they grow up valuing those friendships."

She is so right. In rooms with my close friends, I feel an unbelievable amount of love. There is nothing more anchoring than these women whom I've grown with, shared things with, and cried with for two, three, even four decades. I'm so proud of my long-term friendships, how we've held on to them through the pressures of work, the pressures of family, the pressures of our parents and their health. They've helped me open my heart. I wasn't as capable of that earlier in my life.

Chip Conley told me, "The U-curve of happiness research

shows that the low point in adult life satisfaction is forty-five to fifty. There are all kinds of reasons for this—disappointment with what hasn't been achieved, too many obligations because of being in the 'sandwich generation,' physical health issues starting to crop up. But here's the good news. The U-curve shows that people get happier and happier with each decade after age fifty. And research by Yale's Becca Levy has shown that when we shift our mindset on aging from a negative to a positive, we gain 7.5 years of life. So, maybe midlife is a chrysalis—a time of transformation like the caterpillar to butterfly journey—not a crisis but an awakening.

"This is the time of our lives to imagine what will survive us," Conley says, "the character of our children, that memoir you wrote, the mentee who'll deliver our eulogy, the little dog park that exists in our neighborhood because we helped create it. Our legacy is less about having our name on a building and more about having our imprint on the hearts of the people we've touched and influenced."

In this pro-aging spirit, for my fiftieth birthday, I threw myself a big party. My feeling is, knowing that time is narrowing, we need to keep making good memories. When you know that the window ahead is getting smaller and smaller, why not seize the moment and do what you can to make the rest brilliant? There were forty-five of us—my family, friends I've had for thirty years, and some new friends, too. We had incredible meals and listened to glorious music.

Some of the guests were friends I made when our kids were tiny. Isn't it interesting that we tend to make our closest friends in crucible phases, like when our kids are in preschool and before, when we need that fountain of information? *Are they sleeping through the night? What are you doing about childcare? Are you still breast-feeding?*

Maybe women find one another whenever there's a point of need, when we crave a community to bolster us through new and difficult times. I've made a bunch of new friends through these years of menopause as well, despite thinking I couldn't add more people to my list of close friends.

One of my more poetic friends, Ali, told me that she thinks the culture's fear of menopausal women is really a fear of "women who are no longer malleable, who aren't concerned with the judgments of others anymore, who are reclaiming themselves."

Another says, "Menopause might be 'puberty in reverse,' but the hope is by now there is some understanding of our moods as a welcome consequence of life experience."

I've noticed that even the way women my age walk down the street is different. In our twenties, so many of us feared the predators and felt like prey. When you're aware of too many eyes on you, you shrink your body and don't own space in the same way. Now my friends and I walk with confidence and a lack of self-consciousness.

The activist and author Jodie Patterson said a bad marriage kept her from seeing the ways in which her health was affecting her way of being in the world, but that's all changed: "I now know menopause is a huge factor in how I experience life and interact with those around me. The numbers don't lie: one in three women forty-five to fifty-four years old has been misdiagnosed during menopause. Black women reach menopause 8.5 months earlier than white women and have worse symptoms but are less likely to receive treatment. The question I ask now is: what if women finally became free? Free from misinformation. Free from body shame and guilt. Free from invisibility . . . I love this stage in my life. I've found doctors who care for me and specialize in what I'm experiencing. I sleep more, eat differently, take estrogen, progesterone, and testosterone. I listen to my body and always adjust to complement my constant fluctuations. I've grown better not bitter."

Things are changing. People are sharing more. The stigma surrounding menopause is going away. I believe we're the last generation who will be so deprived of information. Hopefully, our fight has brought a meaningful shift so our daughters will have an easier time.

Dr. Mary Claire Haver told me, "Some of the greatest research coming out right now is looking at ways to extend the life of the ovaries, because they age twice as fast as any other organ in our body. We run out of eggs by about age fifty or fifty-one, and then we're forced to live the rest of our lives without the benefit of our sex hormones. Pretending that that's not going to dramatically affect the course of our health and lives is really silly."

Since that fiftieth birthday party, my friends and I have come to accept that we're older women now, and that, for many of us, being this age is actually better than we were led to believe it would be. Certainly, it's better in so many ways than all the ages up until now. Let's enjoy it!

Some of you might be *in it* right now. I'm also hearing from more and more younger people who are not yet here but trying to prepare. I'd like to tell them that the best things you can do to prepare are what I've come to think of as the five Ts:

TEACHERS: Find people you trust.

TIMELINE: Stay on top of things, but don't let fear drive you.

TENDERNESS: Stay kind toward yourself and others.

TRIBE: Surround yourself with a great community.

TRUTH: Seek the truth in yourself and others.

In your twenties you think you're invincible—other than in the moments when you feel completely vulnerable. In your thirties, you're in a rush—*what am I doing, what's my career, who's my partner, am I going to have kids?* In your forties, you are starting to feel on top of things, but you are required to be all things to all people. And then in your fifties, suddenly you realize everything's . . . maybe fine? Or truly okay. Or at least going to be okay eventually.

"I've come to realize that the selfishness facilitated by divesting domestic and familial responsibilities in maturity can be a super-power if you invest it in self-care," says Mariella Frostrup.

Yes, there are challenges. For instance, nothing makes me feel more irrelevant than technology. If a software update happens, I want to cry for three days. But when I think back on how worthless I felt when I was told I was approaching menopause, I don't recognize that terrified woman. I have forgiven my body. And I've made my peace with relying on my kids to explain memes and trends to me.

I find myself looking back and thinking, *What was I doing? Why did I waste all that time worrying about what other people thought?* I've vowed to do what feels right and to own what I'm good at without apology for whatever time I have left.

Again, Bobbi Brown has been an inspiration to me. She's said that once you reach your sixties you just want to try everything, because why not? The good thing about getting older is that you learn what doesn't matter so much anymore. I used to stress out when my pants were tight or I didn't sleep the night before. Now, I just go with it. No one knows that I'm uncomfortable, so let me stop thinking about it, and let me just drink more water and get through my day, and I'll feel better tomorrow.

"At this age," Bobbi says, "you can enjoy what you have created, and look at your face not as 'Oh, I don't look the same anymore,' but 'This is who I am now.' If you keep yourself limber and strong and healthy, you've got a lot ahead of you. But it requires taking good care of yourself and being very positive in how you speak to yourself."

I agree. I want to keep racking up good experiences, embracing everything I possibly can. I've found so much meaning in surrounding myself with women who demand the truth and who also share their truths. Friendships with history, where we've all experienced extreme highs and lows together. Those are the kind of relationships I rely upon.

Getting to know yourself takes an enormous amount of time

and work. Owning who I am, being vulnerable in my relation-ships, has made me a better partner and friend now than I ever could have been in my twenties and thirties. I don't have time any-more for games or strategy. I think most of the women my age feel the same. There's no room for nonsense.

Menopause can be the true age of liberation for women. If you had kids, they're likely close to leaving or already out of the house. Ideally, you're feeling okay about your romantic relationship, or you've summoned the power to leave and found peace on the other side of divorce. Perhaps you've found someone you like, or you've figured out how to be happy alone. Some of the happiest women I know are single in their fifties and so glad that they can do what-ever they want to do, when they want to do it, without getting anyone else's sign-off.

There are a number of resources you can use in therapy or on-line to interrogate your values—for example, service, physical health, authenticity—and to explore whether you're living by them. One friend of mine swears by Richard Leider's *Power of Purpose* values questionnaires, which you can find online. If you start ex-ploring this terrain, you will find a huge number of potential guides and exercises to help you ask questions about your priorities.

In her book *Find Your Unicorn Space,* Eve Rodsky encourages women to find activities outside their roles as partners, parents, and professionals that light them up. "The oldest tools of the patri-archy are about controlling how women use their time. We have become complicit in our own oppression in a way, where we feel all our time has to go to being good partners, good parents, and good professionals. When I ask, 'What about leisure time?' I find that it is not even part of the vocabulary of a middle-aged woman." Women she spoke to felt guilty for taking even an hour for them-selves.

How do we get out of the cycle of parent, partner, professional? Rodsky believes that there are three principles that allow us to be consistently interested in our own lives: values-based curiosity, sharing yourself with others, and completion (meaning finishing something so you don't live in "a graveyard of unfulfilled dreams").

The empty-nest years can allow us to finally have time to pursue passions and hobbies with greater focus, whether that means reading tarot cards, becoming the family's genealogist, or taking up pottery. According to Rodsky, the key is to focus on your big values and then to find activities that are in line with them. Granny Watts, who plays cards and bingo with a tipple of sherry every night, appears to be having great fun at her nursing home.

Bobbi Brown told me: "One day, a couple of years ago, I was feeling bad because everyone I knew had a hobby. They golfed, they played tennis, they went to plays, they lady-lunched. All I loved doing was working. And then I just stopped. I said, 'All right, Bobbi. Close your eyes. What would be fun?' I've always been the one that at any Bar Mitzvah or wedding is out on the dance floor, and after one cocktail I don't get off. I'll find anyone that will dance with me. So, I found a hip-hop teacher. I just love it."

I realized that I was like Bobbi Brown before she took up dance. My life was work and family and often drawing a blank at press junkets or wondering if I should do something about my jowls. Rodsky pushed me to name my core values beyond family, friends, and health.

I said: authenticity, curiosity, and the need to share to create community or connection.

Rodsky said: "Grab an accountability partner or a success partner and say to yourself, 'Did I get to feel curious this week? If so, did I get to practice community this week? Have I been describing myself as "Zach's mom" or have I been really authentically myself? Did I get a chance to feel curious this week? Did I get a chance to feel true connection this week?'"

You might be well versed in grief now, but ideally, you have found a community to help you through these intense times. You likely don't have that same frenzy to achieve that you had when you were young and didn't know what lay ahead. Best of all, you've fallen on your face so many times by now. The number of humiliations we have been through by this age means we're humbler and more in touch with our own gifts and limitations. We trust that things will swing back.

I spent so much of my life thinking I wasn't smart enough. I learned everything through cumulative experience and finally came to understand that real education doesn't just come from the Ivy League. It comes from falling down and picking yourself back up a million times.

Owning who you are comes from experience, from putting time on the clock. I'm still working at it. But I'm going to stop apologizing. I am done with worrying and trying to make myself smaller, or letting insecurity hold me back. I have too much to do. And too much to enjoy. There is freedom on the other side of the physical turmoil and challenges to your sense of self-worth.

Dr. Jen Gunter is a proponent of the "grandmother hypothesis," the idea that evolution made women outlive their fertility by so many years because they were extremely useful to the community, in particular to their own childbearing children. She told me, "In medical school, I was taught that menopause was a disease. But the grandmother hypothesis is the idea that women actually have an incredibly valuable postreproductive life. Anybody who's had a small child and a helpful set of hands can attest to the value of having somebody around who knows what they're doing. There's research showing that when a mother lives close to her children, her children are likely to have more children."

Some menopausal women will find meaning in taking care of their families, others from starting companies or traveling the world or mentoring young people. So many women have been working their whole lives and are now in management roles.

Every woman will have to figure out what this transition means for her. I've begun to ask: What if the point of menopause is to break up with our former self? It's transitional—you need to leave behind who you were—someone the world considered young, someone who could perhaps get pregnant, someone with far more time ahead of her than behind her. It might not be easy-breezy, but you have to embrace this new person, your present self.

Dr. Carol Tavris told me that the anthropologist Margaret Mead, instead of bemoaning the "change of life" as a phase of endings and decline, celebrated what she called "menopausal zest"—a renewal of energy and opportunity that many women past menopause experience. Women whose children are grown, whose lives are going well and who are in good health, she argued, will find the years past menopause to be a time to experiment, explore, and expand their vistas without being encumbered by the demands of youth and beauty.

Dr. Tavris agrees. "Assuming a woman is not suffering from menopausal symptoms that impair her quality of life, then the years post menopause can absolutely become a time for looking outward. So, get those symptoms taken care of and get out there! Women can use their tremendous energy and potential to make the most of their own lives and the lives of others in our society."

We've ticked the boxes. Some of us didn't check all the ones we wanted and planned to, but maybe we've come to a place of peace with what we have. I believe that comes with time, and it feels good to be at that place. I'd have happily traded the chaos of my twenties and thirties for the life I'm leading in my fifties. I'm more fearless, and more present, and more up for being in the moment. Thank you for coming with me on this journey toward an age of joy, pleasure, and meaning. And please take care of yourself—and remember, you've earned it!

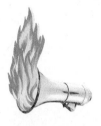

ACKNOWLEDGMENTS

Thanks, first of all, to my grandmothers—proof of how much fulfilling life we can have after middle age—for all the inspiring stories they've shared with me over the years.

I could not have done this without an army of amazing people, starting with my wonderful book agent, Cait Hoyt. I'd also like to thank my manager, Jason Weinberg; my partner in crime, Jason de Beer; and my assistant, Daniel Krane—who all now know more than they ever imagined they'd know about menopause!

I'm grateful to my team for helping connect me with the right publishing house and the right collaborator. Thanks to Ada Calhoun for the endless hours, the attention to detail, and the ability to at once capture my voice and make me sound a thousand times better.

And thank you to my incredible editor, Gillian Blake, for her dedication and hard work, as well as the full team at Crown. Everyone, from the designer Chris Brand, who executed my cover ideas beautifully, the copy editors Terry Deal and Susan M. S. Brown, and the editorial assistant, Amy Li, who has been a joy to work with. Thanks also to our thoughtful fact-checkers, Rachel Stone and Hilary McClellen.

Thank you to the team of doctors who made themselves available because they care deeply about us and share the same goal as me—wanting to see this community thrive, and to calm the waters of misinformation. I want to especially thank Dr. Avrum Bluming,

Dr. Mary Claire Haver, Dr. Somi Javaid, Dr. Sharon Malone, Dr. JoAnn Manson, Dr. Rachel Rubin, Dr. Rocio Salas-Whalen, and Dr. Carol Tavris for lending us your expertise and reviewing chapters of this book. And thanks to my fantastic team at Stripes Beauty, I've learned so much about our need as women to feel seen, heard, and hydrated.

My friends and family have all been saintly through this process. I'm sure I've driven them slightly crazy digging for menopause stories and neurotically tone-checking mine with them over and over again. My goddaughter, Stella Baker, even filled in for a time as my assistant.

My mother continues to inspire me in her sharp wit, bravery, and strength.

Billy: Thank you for your open heart and understanding and for generously letting me tell private stories in this book. You're my gentle, calming, wise other half. Your compassion and curiosity have helped so much with my healing and growth. You're the greatest choice I've ever made other than becoming a mother.

Thanks to Liev for the two most beautiful children and for putting up with me through those hard years of fertility struggles mixed with perimenopausal ups and downs.

To Sasha and Kai: Thank you for testing me and helping me grow every step of the way! All of it has led me to understand myself better and find my sense of purpose. Nothing is more beautiful than getting to watch you becoming yourselves.

Finally, thank you to the community of women out there who have been willing to share their stories and help one another through this time of great challenges and of even greater hope.

So many experts have helped inform my understanding of menopause. Here are a few I'd encourage you to look up as part of your own research.

Dr. Glynis Ablon, aesthetic dermatologist and professor
Dr. Asima Ahmad, ob-gyn and reproductive endocrinologist
Dr. Peter Attia, physician and author of *Outlive: The Science & Art of Longevity*
Minaa B., licensed social worker, mental health educator, and author of *Owning Our Struggles*
Dr. Suzie Bertisch, clinical director of behavorial sleep medicine and assistant professor
Dr. Avrum Bluming, medical oncologist and coauthor of *Estrogen Matters*
Arthur Brooks, social scientist, columnist, and author of *From Strength to Strength*
Bobbi Brown, founder of Jones Road Beauty and Bobbi Brown Cosmetics
Laura Brown, journalist and media personality
Dr. Kelly Casperson, urologist, podcast host, and author of *You Are Not Broken*
Chip Conley, founder of Modern Elder Academy and author of *Learning to Love Midlife*
Dr. Alyssa Dweck, ob-gyn, menopause specialist, and author of *The Complete A to Z for Your V*
Cindy Eckert, entrepreneur and pharmaceutical leader
Dr. Dendy Engelman, dermatologist and Mohs surgeon
Tamsen Fadal, menopause advocate, journalist, author, and podcast host
Dr. Heidi Flagg, ob-gyn and women's health expert
Mariella Frostrup, British journalist and coauthor of *Cracking the Menopause*
Dr. Jennifer Garrison, reproductive longevity and women's health specialist
Dr. Suzanne Gilberg-Lenz, ob-gyn and author of *Menopause Bootcamp*
Dr. Staci Gruber, cognitive and clinical neuroscientist
Dr. Jen Gunter, gynecologist and author of *The Menopause Manifesto* and *The Vagina Bible*

Dan Harris, author of *10% Happier* and host of the *Ten Percent Happier* podcast

Lynn Harris, journalist, novelist, and comedian

Dr. Shelby Harris, sleep specialist and author of *The Women's Guide to Overcoming Insomnia*

Dr. Mary Claire Haver, ob-gyn, culinary medicine specialist, and author of *The New Menopause* and *The Galveston Diet*

Dr. Somi Javaid, ob-gyn and sexual health and menopause specialist and founder of HerMD

Dr. Mohit Khera, professor of urology, sexual medicine expert, and author

Dr. Stacy Lindau, ob-gyn and women's health expert

Elise Loehnen, author and host of the *Pulling the Thread* podcast

Stacy London, stylist

Dr. Sharon Malone, ob-gyn, women's health expert, and author of *Grown Woman Talk*

Dr. JoAnn E. Manson, endocrinologist, professor, and women's health expert

JJ Martin, creator, joy activator, and chief spiritual officer of La DoubleJ

Dr. Wednesday Martin, social scientist and author of *Untrue*

Dr. Leah Millheiser, ob-gyn and sexual wellness specialist

Dr. Laurie Mintz, psychologist, sex therapist, and author of *A Tired Woman's Guide to Passionate Sex*

Dr. Jayne Morgan, cardiologist and women's health expert

Dr. Emily Morse, sex therapist, host of the *Sex with Emily* podcast, and author of *Smart Sex*

Dr. Lisa Mosconi, neuroscientist, educator, and author of *The XX Brain* and *The Menopause Brain*

Emily Nagoski, sex and stress educator and author of *Come As You Are* and *Burnout*

Dr. Rebecca Nelken, ob-gyn and specialist of female pelvic medicine and reconstructive surgeon

Marissa Nelson, marriage and sex therapist and educator

Dr. Robin Noble, ob-gyn and medical director

Dr. Sharon Parish, behavioral medicine and sexual wellness specialist

Dr. Aliza Pressman, developmental psychologist and host of the *Raising Good Humans* podcast

Eve Rodsky, author of *Fair Play* and *Find Your Unicorn Space*

Lauren Roxburgh, author, wellness educator, and body whisperer

Dr. Rachel Rubin, urologist and sexual medicine specialist

Dr. Rocio Salas-Whalen, endocrinologist

Kathryn Schubert, president and CEO of Society for Women's Health Research

Dr. Suzanne Steinbaum, cardiology specialist and women's health expert

Dr. Carol Tavris, social psychologist, feminist, and coauthor of *Estrogen Matters*

Amanda Thebe, fitness expert and author of *Menopocalypse*

Latham Thomas, entrepreneur, author, and professor of gender and sexuality studies

Alisa Volkman, CEO and founder of The Swell

Dr. Ellen Vora, psychiatrist and author of *The Anatomy of Anxiety*

Dr. Amy Wechsler, dermatologist

Dr. Kin Yuen, sleep specialist and professor of behavioral sciences

NOTES

Introduction: What Is Menopause

xvi   **"menopause" was named:** Charles-Pierre-Louis de Gardanne, *De la menopause ou de l'âge critique des femmes* (Lausanne: Méquignon-Marvais), p. 1821.

xix   **two million American women:** Sharon Malone, MD, *Grown Woman Talk: Your Guide to Getting and Staying Healthy* (New York: Crown, 2024), p. 245.

Chapter One: Discomfort Zone

10   **"decreases your risk of UTIs by 50 to 60 percent":** Jasmine Tan-Kim, MD, MAS, Nemi M. Shah, MD, Duy Do, PhD, and Shawn A. Menefee, MD, "Efficacy of Vaginal Estrogen for Recurrent Urinary Tract Infection Prevention in Hypoestrogenic Women," *American Journal of Obstetrics & Gynecology*, August 2023, Vol. 229, Iss. 2, p. 143.

Chapter Two: My Infertility Story

18   **the miscarriage risk is about one in five:** "Miscarriage," *Mayo Clinic*, Mayo Foundation for Medical Education and Research, September 2023, mayoclinic.org/diseases-conditions/pregnancy-loss-miscarriage/symptoms-causes/syc-20354298.

19   **a typical number for a twenty-five-year-old might be 3.0:** "Anti-Mullerian Hormone (AMH) Test: Purpose, Levels & Results," *Cleveland Clinic*, July 2022, my.clevelandclinic.org/health/diagnostics/22681-anti-mullerian-hormone-test.

Chapter Three: Vag of Honor

38 **the Female Sexual Function Index:** "Female Sexual Function Index Questionnaire," in S. D. Reed, K. A. Guthrie, H. Joffe, J. L. Shifren, R. A. Seguin, and E. W. Freeman, "Sexual Function in Nondepressed Women Using Escitalopram for Vasomotor Symptoms: A Randomized Controlled Trial," *Obstetrics and Gynecology,* March 2012, Vol. 119, pp. 527–38.

38 **"the frequency of satisfying sexual events":** Susan R. Davis, Rodney Baber, Nicholas Panay, Johannes Bitzer, Sonia Cerdas Perez, Rakibul M. Islam, Andrew M. Kaunitz, Sheryl A. Kingsberg, Irene Lambrinoudaki, James Liu, Sharon J. Parish, JoAnn Pinkerton, Janice Rymer, James A. Simon, Linda Vignozzi, Margaret E. Wierman, "Global Consensus Position Statement on the Use of Testosterone Therapy for Women," *Maturitas,* September 2019, Vol. 128, pp. 89–93, doi.org/10.1016/j.maturitas.2019.07.001.

Chapter Six: Is Hormone Therapy Safe?

75 **HRT multiplies your risk by about 1.6:** Dominic J. Cirillo, BS; Robert B. Wallace, MD, MSc; Rebecca J. Rodabough, MS; et al., "Effect of Estrogen Therapy on Gallbladder Disease," *JAMA,* January 2005, jamanetwork.com/journals/jama/fullarticle/200193.

Chapter Seven: If I Want to Take Hormones, How Do I Do It?

85 **it affects an enzyme that helps to metabolize medication:** "Grapefruit Juice and Some Drugs Don't Mix," FDA.gov, fda.gov/consumers /consumer-updates/grapefruit-juice-and-some-drugs-dont-mix.

Chapter Eleven: Closet Confidential

138 **dressing for middle age:** Vanessa Friedman, "How Do I Dress for My Menopause Belly and Mood?" *The New York Times,* February 19, 2024.

Chapter Twelve: Menoboss

150 **Approximately 75 percent of women ages forty-five to fifty-five are working:** "Labor Force Participation Rate for Women Highest in the District of Columbia in 2022," *US Bureau of Labor Statistics,* March 7, 2023, bls.gov/opub/ted/2023/labor-force-participation-rate-for-women -highest-in-the-district-of-columbia-in-2022.htm.

Chapter Fifteen: What Does "Family" Look Like Now?

180   **about two-thirds of caregiving:** "Women and Caregiving: Facts and Figures," National Center on Caregiving at Family Caregiver Alliance, www.caregiver.org/resource/women-and-caregiving-facts-and-figures/.

181   **two thousand examples:** Jen Fisher (Host), "Creating Equity at Home and Finding Your Unicorn Space with Eve Rodsky," *WorkWell* podcast, Deloitte, June 12, 2023, deloitte.com/content/dam/Deloitte/us /Documents/about-deloitte/us-workwell-eve-rodsky.pdf.

Chapter Sixteen: Getting the Medical Care You Need

192   **some of the most common problems:** Rachel Nania, "7 Common Health Problems That Can Strike After 50," *AARP*, May 18, 2021, aarp.org/health/conditions-treatments/info-2021/chronic-conditions -after-50.html.

193   **the number-one killer:** "About Women and Heart Disease," CDC, May 15, 2024, cdc.gov/heart-disease/about/women-and-heart-disease .html.

Chapter Seventeen: Closer to Fine

202   **the low point in adult life satisfaction:** Nancy L. Galambos, Harvey J. Krahn, Matthew D. Johnson, Margie E. Lachman, "The U Shape of Happiness Across the Life Course: Expanding the Discussion," *Perspectives on Psychological Science*, July 2020, pp. 898–912.

202   **7.5 years of life:** Caroline Ceniza-Levine, "This Action Can Add 7.5 Years to Your Life Expectancy—3 Ways to Add Career Longevity to Match," *Forbes*, July 2022, forbes.com/sites/carolinecenizalevine/2022 /07/18/this-action-can-add-75-years-to-your-life-expectancy--3-ways -to-add-career-longevity-to-match/.

203   **one in three women:** Harris Poll for Kindra (July 2023), https:// ourkindra.com/blogs/journal/menopause-medical-misdiagnosis.

203   **8.5 months earlier:** S.D. Harlow et al., "Disparities in Reproductive Aging and Midlife Health Between Black and White Women: The Study of Women's Health Across the Nation (SWAN)," *Women's Midlife Health*, Vol. 8, Iss. 3 (2022), doi.org/10.1186/s40695-022-00073-y.

204   **"We run out of eggs by about age fifty or fifty-one":** Emily Mullin, "The Secrets of Aging Are Hidden in Your Ovaries," *Wired*, May 2023, wired.com/story/aging-menopause-longevity/#:~:text=The%20ovary %20is%20a%20time,follicles%20is%20immediate%20and%20unceasing.

209   **"menopausal zest":** Nancy C. Lutkehaus, *Margaret Mead: The Making of an American Icon* (Princeton: Princeton University Press), p. 72.

BIBLIOGRAPHY

If you're ready to do your own deep dive into menopause, here are a few sources I recommend as starting places:

Avrum Bluming and Carol Tavris, *Estrogen Matters* (updated edition, 2024).
Kelly Casperson, *You Are Not Broken: Stop "Should-ing" All Over Your Sex Life* (2022).
Chip Conley, *Learning to Love Midlife* (2024).
Susan Dominus, "Women Have Been Misled About Menopause," *The New York Times Magazine*, February 1, 2023. Updated June 15, 2023.
Jancee Dunn, *Hot and Bothered: What No One Tells You About Menopause* (2023).
Mariella Frostrup and Alice Smellie, *Cracking the Menopause* (2021).
Jen Gunter, *The Menopause Manifesto* (2021) and *The Vagina Bible* (2019).
Mary Claire Haver, *The New Menopause* (2024).
Sharon Malone, *Grown Woman Talk* (2024).
Lisa Mosconi, *The Menopause Brain* (2024).
The Peter Attia Drive Podcast, episode 42, "Avrum Bluming, M.D., and Carol Tavris, Ph.D.: Controversial Topic Affecting All Women—the Role of Hormone Replacement Therapy Through Menopause and Beyond—the Compelling Case for Long-Term HRT and Dispelling the Myth That it Causes Breast Cancer," February 25, 2019.
Kate Rowe-Ham, *Owning Your Menopause* (2024).
Lisa Snowdon, *Just Getting Started: Lessons in Life, Love and Menopause* (2023).
Amanda Thebe, *Menopocalypse* (2020).

INDEX

ABOUT THE AUTHOR

Naomi Watts is a renowned actor and producer. She has received Academy Award nominations for her performances in *21 Grams* and *The Impossible,* and is also known for starring in critically acclaimed projects such as *Mulholland Drive, King Kong,* and, more recently, *Feud: Capote vs. The Swans,* for which she was nominated for a Primetime Emmy Award. She is the founder and chief creative officer of Stripes Beauty, a company dedicated to raising menopause awareness and providing women with education, community, and solutions for a holistic approach to menopause.